P9-DCT-269

FIRST AID
MANUAL

FIRST AID MANUAL

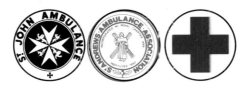

The Authorised Manual of
St. John Ambulance
St. Andrew's Ambulance Association
The British Red Cross Society

1982

Copyright © 1982 by
**The St John Ambulance Association and Brigade,
a Foundation of the Order of St John
St Andrew's Ambulance Association
The British Red Cross Society**

All rights reserved. No part of this publication
may be reproduced, stored in a retrieval system,
or transmitted in any form or by any means, elec-
tronic, mechanical, photocopying, recording or
otherwise, without the prior written permission of
the copyright owners.

Trade edition first published in Great Britain in 1982 by
Dorling Kindersley Limited, 9 Henrietta Street,
Covent Garden, London WC2E 8PS

British Library Cataloguing in Publication Data

St. John Ambulance
The first aid manual.
1.   First aid in illness and injury
I.   Title   II.   St. Andrew's Ambulance
Association   III.   British Red Cross Society
616.02'52   RC87
ISBN 0-86318-000-0
ISBN 0-86318-001-9 Pbk
ISBN 0-86318-007-8 Counter pack

Printed in Italy by A. Mondadori, Verona

FOREWORD

The need for First Aid training is greater than ever.
Populations are growing throughout the world and
the use of mechanical and electrical appliances
and chemicals at home, at work and at leisure,
increases the risk of injury. There is an ever-
increasing demand for First Aid training for personal use in addition to the demand for certificated
First Aiders in industrial, agricultural and commer-
cial establishments.

    The *First Aid Manual* is both an instructional and
a reference book designed to meet the needs of
those interested in First Aid as well as those who
require an acknowledged qualification. It provides
the necessary material for instructional courses.

    Great care has been taken in the preparation of
the fourth edition of the joint *First Aid Manual* to
obtain the views of many of those who render First
Aid and those who see the results of it so as to
make the work as universally acceptable as possible. This has involved consultation with leading
authorities in many fields and the Voluntary
Societies are much indebted for this help. However,
the Joint Revision Committee realises that it is
impossible to produce a definitive work in any tech-
nical field which will secure the immediate and
unreserved approval of all readers and First Aid is
no exception. It is hoped that it will be appreciated
that great care has been taken by the Joint Revision
Committee to evaluate the material in the book to
ensure that as comprehensive and clear a view as
possible is provided, with ample and clear teaching
instructions.

St. John Ambulance
St. Andrew's Ambulance Association
The British Red Cross Society

CONTENTS

HOW TO USE THIS BOOK

The joint *First Aid Manual* contains all the information which is necessary for standard First Aid courses. The Voluntary Societies will, after careful assessment of the theoretical and practical knowledge of each candidate following a recognised course of instruction, award First Aid certificates.

The information in the *First Aid Manual* is divided into three main sections and each section is denoted by different page borders. The major First Aid techniques, those which are vital to save lives, are contained in one chapter at the front of the book; these pages are marked by a wide, red border. Here you will find the techniques for resuscitation and the control of bleeding.

The main section of the book, marked by thin red page borders, contains chapters which deal generally with situations such as *Action at an Emergency* and *Procedure at Major Incidents*, and others which deal specifically with conditions relating to the major classifications such as *Asphyxia*, *Wounds and Bleeding*, *Circulatory Disorders* and *Unconsciousness*. In each case the condition is defined and the possible symptoms and signs and the recommended treatment are described. The treatments are all set out in simple step-by-step form and are accompanied by descriptive illustrations to make them easier to follow. It is also important to realise that all the symptoms and signs listed as part of any condition do not necessarily occur in the order given and may not all be present in every condition.

Towards the end of the book are two chapters — *Dressings and Bandages* and *Handling and Transport* — which contain information relevant to all conditions. These chapters are denoted by wide, grey page borders.

As a general principle, information on the structure and function of parts of the body have been included in some of the chapters in order to aid understanding of the treatment described.

The chapter on *Emergency Childbirth* at the end of the book is included to provide the necessary information should the emergency arise without normal facilities being immediately available. This subject, however, does *not* form part of a Standard First Aid course and is therefore *not* required for any examination purposes.

The *First Aid Manual* can be used as a guideline for treatment by the untrained. However, the life-saving techniques of Artificial Ventilation and External Chest Compression should *not* be used until you have received proper instruction from a trained instructor.

THE PRINCIPLES AND PRACTICE OF FIRST AID

First Aid is the skilled application of accepted principles of treatment on the occurrence of any injury or sudden illness, using facilities or materials available to you at the time. It is the approved method of treating a casualty until placed, if necessary in the care of a doctor or removed to hospital.

Why it is Given

First Aid treatment is given to a casualty:
● To preserve life.
● To prevent the condition worsening.
● To promote recovery.

The Responsibility of the First Aider

Because of the frequency and serious nature of many accidents, the role of the First Aider is very important.

In the management of a casualty, your responsibility as a First Aider is to:
● Assess the situation.
● Identify the disease or condition from which the casualty is suffering (diagnosis).
● Give immediate, appropriate and adequate treatment, bearing in mind that a casualty may have more than one injury and that some casualties will require more urgent attention than others.
● Arrange, without delay, for the disposal of a casualty to a doctor, hospital or home, according to the seriousness of the condition.

Your responsibility ends when the casualty is handed over to the care of a doctor, a nurse or other appropriate person. You should not leave the incident until you have made your report to whoever takes charge and have ascertained whether you could be of any further help.

Definitions

Medical aid indicates treatment by a doctor at a hospital or surgery.
First Aider is the term which describes any person who has received a certificate from an authorised training body indicating that he or she is qualified to render First Aid . It was first used in 1894 by the Voluntary First Aid Organisations.

First Aid certificates issued by St. John Ambulance, St. Andrew's Ambulance Association and the British Red Cross Society are awarded to candidates who have attended a course of theoretical and practical work and who have passed a professionally supervised examination.

The certificate awarded is only valid for three years thus ensuring First Aiders are:
● Highly trained.
● Regularly examined.
● Kept up-to-date in knowledge and skill.

MAJOR FIRST AID TECHNIQUES

Skilled First Aiders can save lives by maintaining a casualty's vital needs. Commonly abbreviated as ABC these needs are:

A An open *Airway*
B Adequate *Breathing*
C Sufficient *Circulation*

For life to continue, a person must be able to take oxygen into the lungs. This will, in turn, be distributed throughout the body by the blood. While it is possible for some parts of the body to survive for a time without oxygen, some organs are very quickly affected — vital nerve cells in the brain can die after only three minutes.

The three emergency situations where a casualty is especially at risk because of interference with vital needs are listed below. (The order may vary according to the situation.)

● Lack of breathing and/or heartbeat.
● Severe bleeding.
● A state of unconsciousness which, as it develops, is likely to interfere with the open airway and eventually breathing.

The techniques in this chapter are:

For AIRWAY
Opening the airway to allow unobstructed passage of fresh air to the lungs.

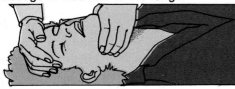

The *Recovery Position* to help maintain an open airway so preventing the unconscious casualty becoming asphyxiated.

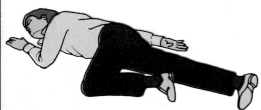

For BREATHING
Artificial Ventilation to get air into the lungs of a casualty who has stopped breathing.

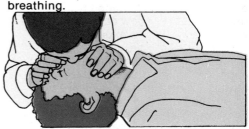

For CIRCULATION
External Chest Compression to apply pressure on the chest to compress the heart and so pump blood through the arteries to the vital organs.

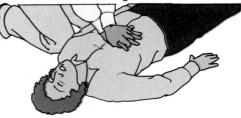

Controlling severe bleeding to prevent or minimise serious blood loss so that a casualty's circulation can be maintained.

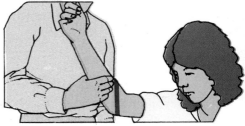

It is important to practise these techniques under trained supervision as no text book description is a substitute for practical knowledge and experience.

You must know how the body functions during respiration and circulation so that you can apply these special techniques.

RESPIRATION

Oxygen is vital to support life. The aim of breathing is to transfer oxygen from the air to the lungs where it can be picked up by the blood and circulated throughout the body, and to allow carbon dioxide, a waste product, to be expelled.

When you breathe, air is drawn in at the nose or mouth and sucked down a main airway, the windpipe (trachea), through smaller passages (bronchi), and finally reaches air sacs (alveoli) in the lungs where an exchange of gases is made. In these small sacs, oxygen is picked up by the blood and carbon dioxide is given up by the blood to be breathed out.

Air is a mixture of gases: 21% of it is oxygen. Only 5% of the oxygen is used up in breathing, so that when we exhale, we breathe out 16% in addition to a small amount of carbon dioxide. The amount of oxygen breathed out is therefore adequate to resuscitate another person.

In the mouth and throat, food and air share the same passage, but at the top of the main airway is the voice box (larynx). This structure not only serves as the organ of speech but also acts as a valve which closes whenever you swallow, thus preventing the inhalation of food or drink. However, in an unconscious person, this protective mechanism works less well and becomes increasingly ineffective as unconsciousness deepens.

The Respiratory System

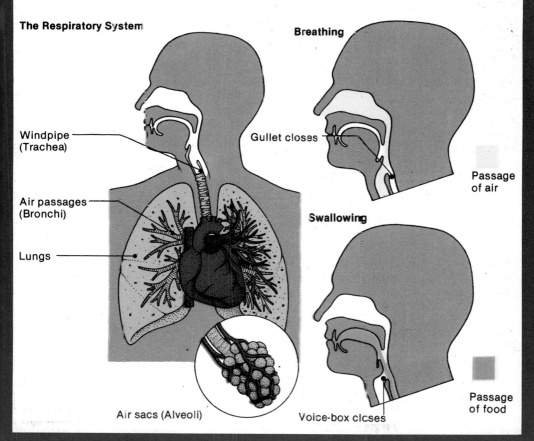

Windpipe (Trachea)

Air passages (Bronchi)

Lungs

Air sacs (Alveoli)

Breathing

Gullet closes

Passage of air

Swallowing

Voice-box closes

Passage of food

HOW WE BREATHE

Breathing is divided into three phases: breathing-in (inspiration), breathing-out (expiration) and pause. When you breathe in, the chest muscles pull the ribs upwards allowing the chest to expand in width and height. The diaphragm, a strong muscular partition which separates the chest cavity from the abdominal cavity, contracts and flattens increasing the chest's capacity from below. This combined action causes air to be sucked into the lungs so that the exchange of gases can take place. When breathing out, the diaphragm and the rib muscles relax and resume their position at rest. A short pause follows before the cycle starts all over again.

In normal respiration some residual air is left in the lungs so that circulating blood always has some oxygen available.

A respiratory centre in the brain determines the rate and depth of breathing: the average adult normally breathes 16 to 18 times per minute, and children and infants breathe 20 to 30 times per minute. This rate often increases during stress, exercise, injury or illness. The heart rate will increase accordingly to carry the extra oxygen around the body.

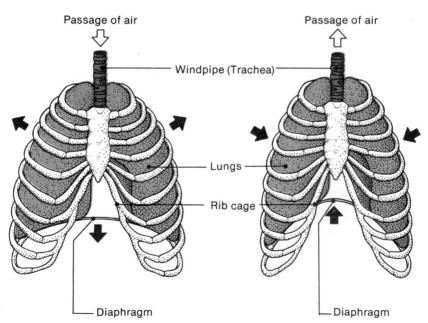

Inhalation

Exhalation

Passage of air

Passage of air

Windpipe (Trachea)

Lungs

Rib cage

Diaphragm

Diaphragm

Key

Black arrows indicate the direction of movement of the rib cage and diaphragm during breathing.

White arrows indicate the passage of air during breathing.

HOW OXYGEN IS CIRCULATED IN THE BLOOD

Oxygen is carried around the body by the red cells in the blood (see p. 88). Blood is circulated in a continuously repeated cycle by the contraction-relaxation movement of the heart. Each time the heart muscle contracts, blood is forced out of the pumping chambers of the heart; when the muscle relaxes, replacement blood pours into its collecting chambers. In the average adult at rest the heart "beats" about 72 times per minute.

Deoxygenated blood flows back from the tissues into two main veins, and then into the right side of the heart. It is then forced out of the heart to the lungs where the exchange of gases takes place. The oxygenated blood returns to the left side of the heart and is then "pumped" out again into the main artery from where it is distributed to all parts of the body (see *Blood and the Circulation* p. 26). Valves in the heart ensure that blood continues to flow in the right direction.

The oxygenated red blood cells give the blood its bright red colour; blueness (cyanosis) arises when the blood is low in oxygen; pallor results from a lack of blood in the skin. These colour changes are especially noticeable in the lips, earlobes and nail beds.

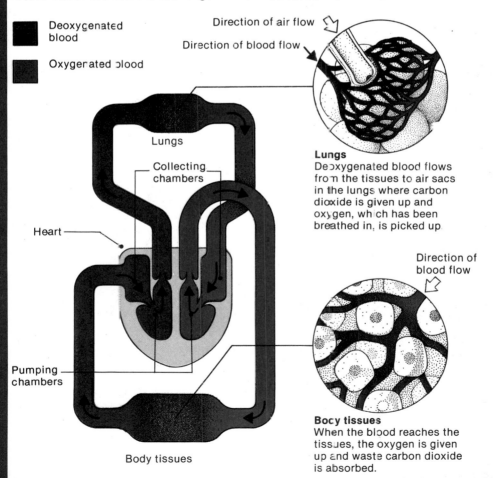

Deoxygenated blood

Oxygenated blood

Direction of air flow

Direction of blood flow

Lungs

Collecting chambers

Heart

Pumping chambers

Body tissues

Lungs
Deoxygenated blood flows from the tissues to air sacs in the lungs where carbon dioxide is given up and oxygen, which has been breathed in, is picked up.

Direction of blood flow

Body tissues
When the blood reaches the tissues, the oxygen is given up and waste carbon dioxide is absorbed.

RESUSCITATION

If a casualty is not breathing and if the heart is not beating, it is vital that you take over respiration and circulation so that the flow of oxygen to the brain is maintained. Remember your ABCs. First, ensure an open *airway*; second, *breathe* for the casualty by inflating the lungs and oxygenating the blood (Artificial Ventilation); third, *circulate* the blood by compressing the chest (External Chest Compression).

The quick and efficient use of Artificial Ventilation, if necessary combined with External Chest Compression, should prevent further deterioration of the casualty's condition and preserve life until more skilled help is available. Resuscitation should be attempted even if you are in doubt about whether a casualty is capable of being revived. You should always continue until: spontaneous breathing and pulse are restored; another qualified person takes over; a doctor assumes responsibility for the casualty; or you are exhausted and unable to continue.

Checking Breathing

In order to find out whether a casualty is breathing, place your ear above the casualty's mouth and look along the chest and abdomen. If the casualty is breathing you will hear and feel any breaths and see movement along the chest and abdomen. A casualty who has stopped breathing will almost certainly be unconscious: it is not always easy to discern the exact moment that a casualty stops breathing.

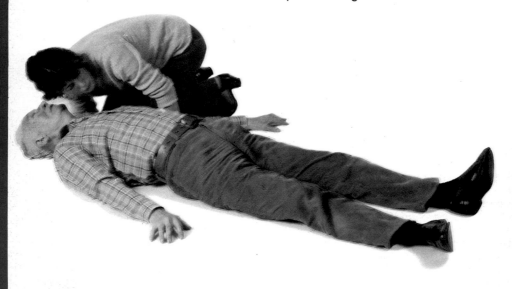

Opening the Airway

If a casualty is unconscious, the airway may be narrowed or blocked making breathing difficult or impossible. This occurs for several reasons: the head may tilt forward narrowing the air passage; muscular control in the throat will be lost, which may allow the tongue to slip back and block the air passage; and, because the reflexes are impaired, saliva or vomit may lie in the back of the throat blocking the airway. Any of these situations can lead to the death of the casualty so it is imperative that you establish a clear airway immediately.

With an open airway a casualty may begin breathing spontaneously. If the casualty does begin breathing, place in the Recovery Position (see p. 24). If the casualty still does not breathe, you will have to begin resuscitation.

Method

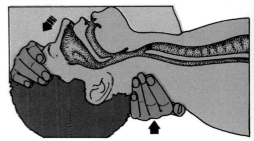

1 Place one hand under the casualty's neck and your other hand on the forehead and tilt the head backwards. This will extend the head and neck and open the air passage.

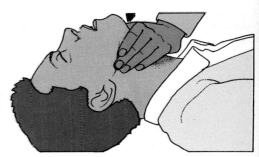

2 Transfer your hand from the neck and push the chin upwards. The tilted jaw will lift the tongue forward, clear of the airway.

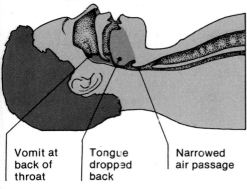

Vomit at back of throat | Tongue dropped back | Narrowed air passage

Clearing the Airway

In the Open Airway Position any foreign matter such as vomit, loose teeth or dentures, or food that can be seen or felt should be removed if possible. To achieve this, turn the casualty's head to the side; hook your first two fingers and sweep round inside the mouth. But, *do not spend time searching for hidden obstructions*.

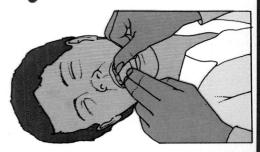

Breathing for the Casualty

The most efficient way you can breathe for a casualty is to transfer air from your own lungs into the casualty's, by blowing into them through the mouth (Mouth-to-Mouth Ventilation). Sometimes, however, this is not possible in which case you may have to use one of the manual methods (see pp. 30 – 32).

MOUTH-TO-MOUTH VENTILATION

The air we exhale contains about 16% oxygen which is more than is needed to sustain life (see *Respiration* p. 11). In Mouth-to-Mouth Ventilation you blow air from your lungs into the casualty's mouth or nose (or mouth and nose together in a child) to fill the casualty's lungs. When you take your mouth away, the casualty will breathe out as the elastic chest wall resumes its shape at rest. Mouth-to-Mouth Ventilation enables you to watch the casualty's chest for movement, indicating that the lungs are being filled or that the casualty is breathing again naturally, and to observe changes in the casualty's colour (see p. 21).

Mouth-to-Mouth Ventilation can be used by First Aiders of any age and in most circumstances. It is easiest to carry out if the casualty is lying on the back, but it should be started immediately whatever position the casualty happens to be in. The first four inflations must be given swiftly. The casualty may start breathing again at any stage but may need assistance until breathing settles down into a normal rate.

The only occasion on which Mouth-to-Mouth Ventilation *must not* be used is in some cases of poisoning where contamination around the casualty's mouth can affect the rescuer. It may also be unsuitable if there are serious facial injuries, if there is recurrent vomiting or if the casualty is pinned face-down.
NB Future references to Mouth-to-Mouth Ventilation include Mouth-to-Nose and Mouth-to-Mouth-and-Nose.

Assisting the Casualty's Circulation

It is pointless continuing Artificial Ventilation if the casualty's heart is not beating, because the oxygenated blood will not be circulating. After the first four ventilations you must check carefully to see whether the heart is beating (see below). Always remember that while it is sometimes acceptable to assist breathing which s failing, the heart action is easily upset, so *never attempt External Chest Compression if the heart is beating, even faintly.*

EXTERNAL CHEST COMPRESSION

Contractions can be simulated in a non-beating heart by compressing the chest. By pressing down on to the lower third of the breastbone you increase the pressure inside the chest thus driving blood out of the heart and into the arteries. When you release the pressure, the chest returns to its normal position and blood flows back along the veins and refills the heart as it expands.

External Chest Compression is *always* preceded, and accompanied, by Artificial Ventilation. To be effective, it must be carried out with the casualty lying on a firm surface. As soon as you feel a spontaneous pulse returning to the carotid artery stop External Chest Compression immediately, but carry on with Artificial Ventilation on its own, if it is necessary.

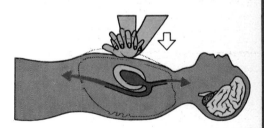

Checking for Heartbeat

Before commencing External Chest Compression it is very important that you establish that there is no heartbeat. Although the casualty may be blue around the lips (cyanosed) if the heart is not pumping blood to the surface, the only reliable way of establishing a lack of heartbeat is to check the pulse at the neck (carotid pulse). This pulse can be felt at the neck in the hollow between the voice box and the adjoining muscle. (The pulse at the wrist is an unreliable indication). It must be checked again after the first minute and then every three minutes thereafter. It will only return spontaneously if the heart is beating.

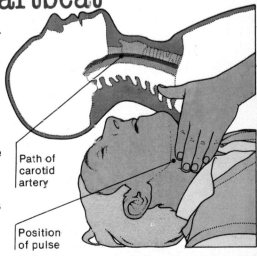

Path of carotid artery

Position of pulse

Mouth-to-Mouth Ventilation

This is the preferred method of Artificial Ventilation in ALL cases where a casualty is not breathing (except for the few listed on p. 16). If the mouth cannot be used, satisfactory ventilation can be achieved through the nose (Mouth-to-Nose) or through the mouth and nose in small children and infants (Mouth-to-Mouth-and-Nose).

NB Give the first four inflations as soon as possible; do not spend time looking for hidden obstructions.

Method

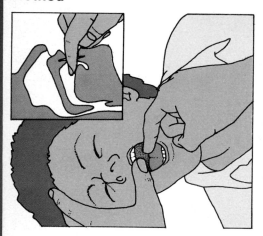

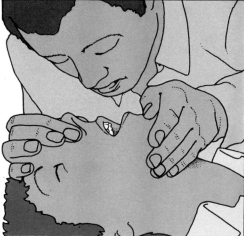

1 Remove any obvious obstructions over the face or constrictions around the neck. Open the airway (see p. 15) and remove any debris seen in the mouth or the throat.

2 Open your mouth wide, take a deep breath, pinch the nostrils together with your fingers and seal your lips around the mouth. (For Mouth-to-Nose, close the casualty's mouth with your thumb and seal your lips around the casualty's nose.)

Mouth-to-nose ventilation

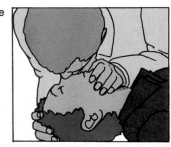

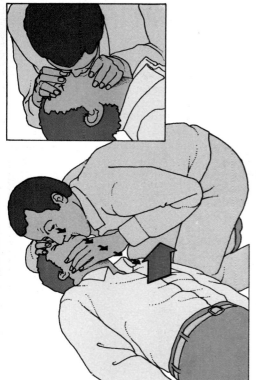

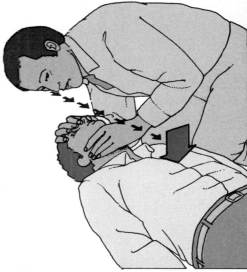

3 Looking along the chest, blow into the casualty's lungs until you can see the chest rise to maximum expansion.

NB If the casualty's chest fails to rise, first assume the airway is not fully open. Adjust the position of the head and jaw and try again. If there is still no ventilation, the airway may be blocked, and you will have to treat for *Choking* (see p. 51).

4 Remove your mouth well away from the casualty's and breathe out any excess air. Watch the chest fall and take in fresh air. Repeat inflation.
Give the first four inflations as quickly as possible without waiting for complete lung deflation between breaths.

5 Check the casualty's pulse to make sure the heart is beating (see *Checking for Heartbeat* p. 17).

If the heart is beating normally, continue to give inflations at normal breathing rate (16 – 18 times per minute) until natural breathing is restored, assisting it when necessary and adjusting it to the casualty's breathing rate. When the casualty is breathing normally, place in the Recovery Position (see p. 24).

If the heart is not beating you must perform External Chest Compression immediately (see overleaf).

External Chest Compression

If Mouth-to-Mouth Ventilation by itself is unsuccessful and the casualty's heart stops, or has stopped beating, you must perform External Chest Compression in conjunction with Mouth-to-Mouth Ventilation. This is because without the heart to circulate the blood, oxygenated blood cannot reach the casualty's brain.

Method

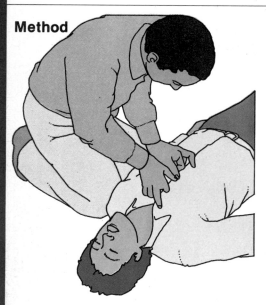

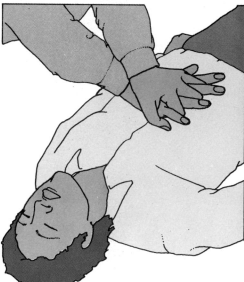

1 Lay the casualty on the back on a firm surface. Kneel alongside the casualty facing the chest and in line with the heart. Locate the lower half of the breastbone; find the sternal notch at the top and the intersection of the rib margins at the bottom. Place your thumbs midway between these two landmarks to find the centre.

2 Place the heel of one hand on the centre of lower half of the breast-bone, keeping your fingers off the ribs. Cover this hand with the heel of your other hand and lock your fingers together.

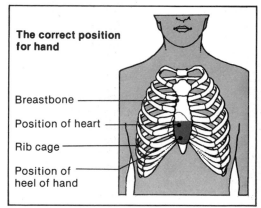

The correct position for hand

Breastbone

Position of heart

Rib cage

Position of heel of hand

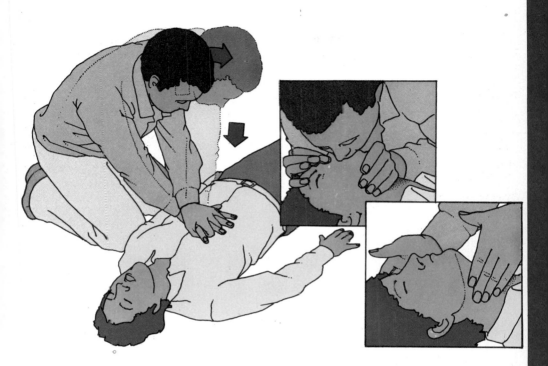

3 Keep your arms straight and rock forwards until your arms are vertical. Press down on the lower half of the breastbone (about 4 to 5 cm/1½ to 2 in for the average adult). Rock backwards to release pressure. Complete fifteen compressions at the rate of eighty compressions per minute. (To find the correct speed, count one and two and three, and so on.)

Checking for Response

When resuscitation is successful, the carotid pulse will return. Look at the casualty's face and lips. The colour will improve as blood containing oxygen begins to circulate. When the casualty is not breathing, the normal colour turns blue (cyanosis).

4 Move back to the casualty's head and re-open the airway. Seal the airway and give two breaths of Mouth-to-Mouth Ventilation.

5 Continue with fifteen compressions followed by two full ventilations, repeating heart check after the first minute. Thereafter, check heartbeat after every twelve cycles or three minutes.

6 As soon as the heartbeat returns, stop compressions immediately. Continue Mouth-to-Mouth Ventilation until natural breathing is restored, assisting it when necessary, and adjusting it to the casualty's rate. Place the casualty in the Recovery Position (see p. 24).

Resuscitation with Two First Aiders

When two First Aiders are present, one should take charge and maintain the open airway, perform Mouth-to-Mouth Ventilation and check heartbeat; the other should perform External Chest Compression. If resuscitation is prolonged, the First Aiders can change places to reduce the strain, and it may be easier if they work on opposite sides of the body.

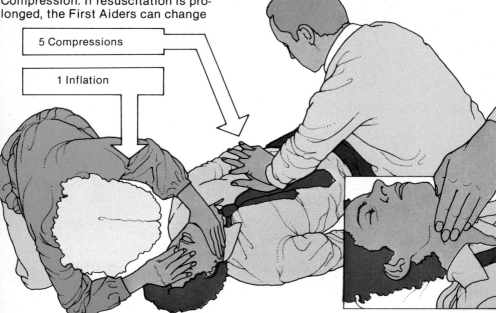

5 Compressions

1 Inflation

1 One First Aider takes up a position at the casualty's head, the other kneels alongside the casualty level with the middle of the chest.

2 The First Aider at the head immediately opens the airway, gives the first four inflations and checks for heartbeat (see p. 17). If it is absent, the other First Aider should give five chest compressions.

3 Resuscitation then continues with the First Aider at the head opening the airway and giving a *single* inflation followed by the other giving five compressions. This is performed continuously at a rate of sixty compressions per minute until the heartbeat is found. (To find the correct speed, count 1001, 1002, and so on.)
Heartbeat check must be carried out after the first minute and then after every three minutes or twelve cycles.

NB the operator at the head gives the inflation on the upstroke of the fifth compression so that there is no pause.

Resuscitation for Children

The techniques for resuscitating youths and older children are the same as for adults (see pp. 18 – 21), but they must be done slightly faster and with lighter pressure. For children and infants use the techniques described below and place your hand over the *centre* of the breastbone for External Chest Compression.

FOR CHILDREN

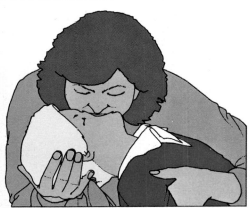

1 Perform Mouth-to-Mouth Ventilation by sealing your lips around the child's mouth and nose and breathing gently into the lungs at a rate of 20 breaths per minute. Check for heartbeat after giving the first four inflations.

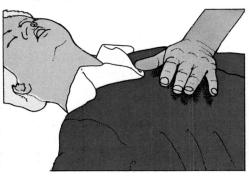

2 Perform External Chest Compression with light pressure using *one hand only*. Press at a rate of 100 compressions per minute to a depth of 2.5 to 3.5 cm (1 to 1.5 in) with fifteen compressions to two ventilations.

FOR INFANTS AND SMALL CHILDREN

When resuscitating infants give very gentle puffs and use very light pressure with two fingers only; apply at a rate of fifteen compressions to two ventilations.

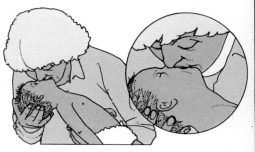

1 Perform Mouth-to-Mouth Ventilation by sealing your lips around the baby's *mouth and nose* and puffing gently into the lungs at a rate of 20 breaths per minute. Check for heartbeat after giving the first four inflations.

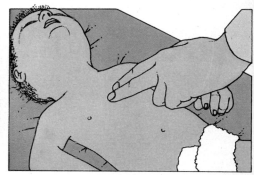

2 Perform External Chest Compression with *two fingers* pressing at a rate of 100 times per minute to a depth of 1.5 to 2.5 cm (0.5 to 1 in).

The Recovery Position

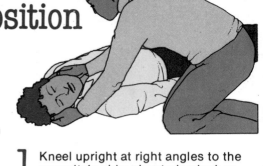

Unconscious casualties who are breathing and whose hearts are beating should be placed in the *Recovery Position*. This position ensures that a casualty maintains an open airway, that the tongue cannot fall to the back of the throat, that the head and neck will remain in the extended position so that the air passage is widened, and that any vomit or other fluid in the casualty's mouth will drain freely. The position of the casualty's limbs provides the necessary stability to keep the body propped in a safe and comfortable position. Depending upon the casualty's injuries or condition, you may have to modify the technique in order to avoid causing further damage to injuries.

The Recovery Position may not be an ideal position initially if you are examining a casualty or for treatment of a spine injury. However, it *must* be used immediately if a casualty's breathing becomes difficult or noisy and is not relieved by opening the airway or if a casualty has to be left unattended (an unusual event).

Illustrated opposite is the sequence of turning a casualty who is lying on the back; not all these steps will be necessary if the casualty is lying on the side or front. If the casualty is wearing spectacles, these should be removed before turning the head to avoid eye injuries.

1 Kneel upright at right angles to the casualty's side, about nine inches away and level with the chest. Turn the head towards you and tilt it back keeping the jaw forward in the Open Airway Position (see p. 15).

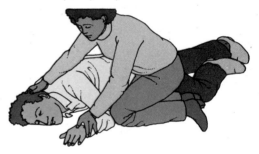

4 Still supporting the casualty's body against your knees, re-adjust the head to ensure that the airway is open.

5 Bend the casualty's uppermost arm into a convenient position to support the upper body.

FOR A HEAVY CASUALTY

You may have to use both hands to turn a heavy casualty. Grasp the clothing at the shoulders and hips and pull the casualty so that the body is against your thighs.

If bystanders are present, one may support the head while you do the turning. Alternatively, get them to help by kneeling beside you and by pulling alongside you with both hands at the hips while you pull the shoulders and support the head. It may be necessary for them to face you and push the casualty towards you as you pull.

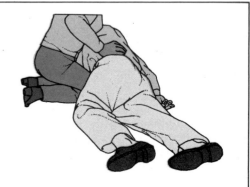

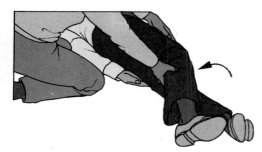

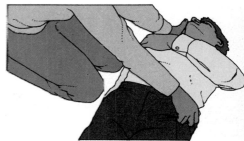

2 Place the casualty's arm nearest to you by the side. Place the casualty's hand under the buttock, palm upwards if possible. Bring the other forearm over the front of the chest. Holding the far leg under the knee or ankle bring it towards you and cross it over the near leg.

3 Protect and support the casualty's head with one hand. With the other hand, grasp the clothing at the hip furthest from you and pull the casualty quickly towards you. Support the casualty on the side against your knees.

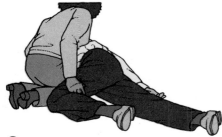

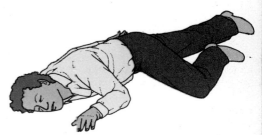

6 Bend the casualty's uppermost leg at the knee to bring the thigh well forward to support the lower body.

7 Carefully pull the other arm out from under the casualty, working from the shoulder down. Leave it lying parallel to the casualty to prevent the casualty rolling on to the back.

MODIFICATIONS

Do not follow the above method where there are fractures to the upper or lower body, when the casualty is lying in a confined space or if it is not possible to use the bent limbs as props. In such cases, the Recovery Position can be maintained by laying a rolled blanket down the front of the body. This method can also be used to transport a casualty on a stretcher in the Recovery Position.

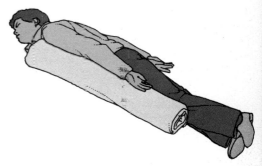

BLOOD AND THE CIRCULATION

There are approximately 6 litres (10 pints) of blood in the normal adult's circulatory system. Blood carries oxygen and other nutrients to the tissues, and carbon dioxide and other waste products away from them. It flows through a network of flexible tubes called blood vessels.

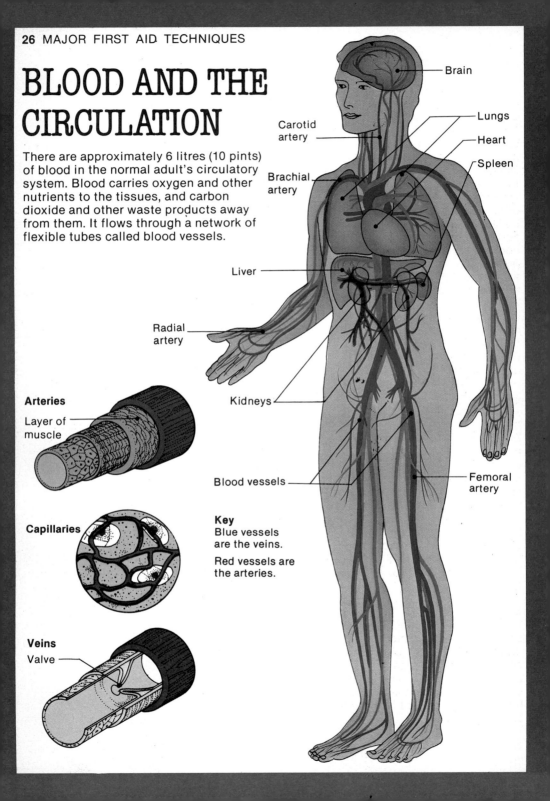

Brain

Carotid artery

Lungs

Heart

Spleen

Brachial artery

Liver

Radial artery

Kidneys

Arteries

Layer of muscle

Blood vessels

Femoral artery

Capillaries

Key
Blue vessels are the veins.

Red vessels are the arteries.

Veins

Valve

Arteries carry blood away from the heart. They are the strongest of the blood vessels and their walls contain elastic and muscular tissue. As the blood is forced along the arteries by the action of the heart, the muscular wall expands and then returns to its normal size. This wave of pressure is called the *pulse* and it can be felt wherever an artery is close to the surface and can be pressed against a bone, at the neck or wrist, for example (see p. 89). Arteries divide becoming smaller and thinner as they reach the tissues until they become capillaries.

Capillaries are very small blood vessels, consisting only of a thin layer of cells through which the exchange of fluids and gases to and from the tissue cells of the body can be made. Having done this, the tiny capillaries gradually join up and become veins.

Veins carry blood back to the heart. Smaller veins unite, gradually becoming larger until they end in two large veins which return the blood to the right collecting chamber of the heart. Veins have no muscular layer, and they rely on "back" pressure and the squeezing action of the body muscles to make blood flow through them. Because of this, veins in the lower part of the body have one-way "cup-like" valves which help to control the flow of blood back to the heart.

Severe Bleeding

When you cut yourself you bleed because pressure inside the blood vessels forces blood out. In arterial bleeding, bright red-coloured blood pumps out in time with the heart; in venous bleeding, the blood is a darker red and gushes out with less pressure; in capillary bleeding, blood oozes out.

The body contains certain inbuilt mechanisms to slow down or stop bleeding spontaneously. When a wound occurs the cut ends of a blood vessel contract to reduce the loss of blood and blood pressure falls. Blood clots form and plug up damaged vessels. The more slowly blood flows from a wound, the easier it is for a clot to form; the faster blood flows, the more likely it is that any clots will be washed away.

The Dangers of Blood Loss

Normally the loss of a pint of blood in an adult is barely noticeable (e.g., a donor) but by the time that three pints, or about a third of blood volume is lost, the results can be serious because there is not enough left to provide a sufficient flow around the body. If you do not act quickly to stop severe bleeding there is a danger that shock, and even loss of the casualty's life, may result.

The symptoms and signs of severe blood loss are due partly to the blood loss itself, and partly to the body's reaction to that loss; they may not all be apparent in every casualty. The face and lips become pale and the skin feels cold and clammy as the vessels which supply blood to the skin constrict in order to divert blood to the vital organs. To compensate for the blood loss, the pulse becomes faster, but weaker. If bleeding is prolonged, there may be a reduction in the flow of blood to the brain, resulting in blurring of vision, giddiness, clouding of consciousness and fainting. In addition, the casualty may become anxious, restless and talkative for the same reason. (See also *Shock* p. 90.)

Blood loss can also cause a feeling of thirst resulting from the body's natural urge to replace lost fluid, and a hunger for air to replace lost oxygen.

You should act quickly to stop any bleeding but, urgently if:
- A large amount of blood is being lost.
- The bleeding appears to be arterial — bright red and spurting regularly.
- The bleeding has continued for an abnormally long time.

Controlling Blood Loss

The principle of controlling blood loss is to restrict the blood flow to the wound and therefore encourage clotting. This is done in two ways — by *pressure* and by *elevation*. There are two kinds of pressure: direct pressure over the wound and indirect pressure on the artery which supplies the area. Direct pressure must always be applied first; only use indirect pressure if this fails or is difficult.

Direct Pressure

In order to stop bleeding without interfering with the rest of circulation, you should apply pressure directly on a wound immediately. This direct pressure flattens the blood vessels in the area and helps to slow down the flow of blood, so that clots can form. Pressure has to be maintained for five to fifteen minutes because it takes time to halt the flow of blood. If there is a foreign body embedded in the wound, pressure has to be applied alongside it.

If possible, you should also raise the injured part and support it in this position. This will slow down the flow of blood by lowering the local blood pressure.

Method

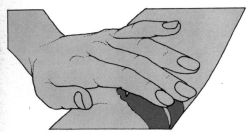

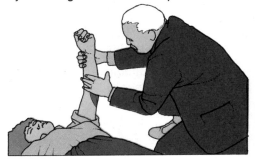

1 Apply direct pressure on the wound with thumb and/or fingers.

2 Lay the casualty down in a suitable and comfortable position. Raise the injured part as far as possible and support it.

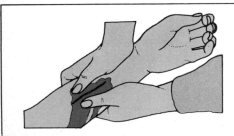

If the wound is large, squeeze the sides of the wound together gently but firmly and maintain pressure.

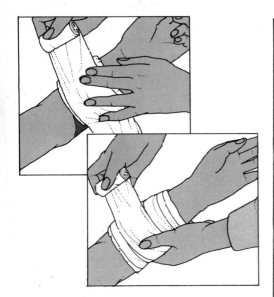

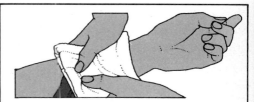

If no suitable dressing is available, place a piece of gauze over the wound, cover it with a pad of cotton wool and bandage firmly. An improvised dressing can be made from any suitable clean material (see p. 175). Immobilise injured part (see *Fractures* pp. 106 – 127).

3 Place a sterile, unmedicated dressing over the wound, making sure it extends well beyond the edges of the wound. Press it down firmly and secure with a bandage tied firmly enough to control bleeding, but not so tight as to cut off circulation (see p. 178).

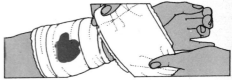

If bleeding continues, apply further dressings or pads and bandage firmly. Do not remove the original dressing as this may disturb clots and re-start the bleeding.

Indirect Pressure

If bleeding cannot be controlled by direct pressure or if it is impossible to apply direct pressure successfully (for example, if there are severe lacerations), you may be able to control it by applying indirect pressure at the appropriate pressure point. However, this method can only be used to control arterial bleeding.

A pressure point is the place where you can compress an artery against an underlying bone to flatten it and prevent the flow of blood beyond that point. However, since this cuts off the supply of blood to the tissues of the entire limb, *this method should only be used as a last resort and must not be applied for longer than fifteen minutes*.

There are two pressure points used to control severe bleeding, one is on the *brachial* artery in the arm, and the other is on the *femoral* artery in the thigh.

The brachial artery runs along the inner side of the upper arm between the muscles and its course roughly follows the seam of the sleeve. To apply pressure, pass your fingers under the casualty's arm and slide them between the muscles. Press upwards and inwards pushing the artery against the bone.

The femoral artery passes into the lower limb at a point corresponding to the centre of the fold of the groin and runs along the inside of the thigh. To apply pressure, lay the casualty down with knee bent. Locate the artery in the groin and press it against the rim of the pelvis with your fist or the heel of your hand.

MANUAL METHODS OF ARTIFICIAL VENTILATION

There will be occasions in which Mouth-to-Mouth Ventilation cannot be used, and these are:

● If there are severe facial injuries involving both the casualty's mouth and nose.
● If the casualty is trapped in a face-downwards position.
● If there is recurrent vomiting.
● Cases of poisoning where any contamination around the casualty's mouth can affect the First Aider.
There are two manual methods which can be used — the *Holger Nielsen* and the *Silvester* — but they are not as efficient as Mouth-to-Mouth. The Silvester method cannot be used if the casualty is trapped face-down or if there is recurrent vomiting, and neither method can be used if there are serious injuries to the arms or the chest.

Both methods involve pushing on the chest from the front or back, to force air out of the lungs, then moving the casualty's arms upwards and outwards to expand the chest and produce inspiration.

As with normal resuscitation, a much lighter pressure and faster rate will be necessary when performing these methods of resuscitation on children.

CHECKING FOR RESPONSE
If resuscitation is successful the casualty's colour will improve (see p. 21). If no improvement is noticed after the first four ventilations, there may be an obstruction in the airway (see p. 51).

The Holger Nielsen Method

This is the next preferred method of Artificial Ventilation after Mouth-to-Mouth because it maintains the open airway while the casualty is in a face downwards position. However, while the casualty is in this position you cannot perform External Chest Compression nor can you easily check for heartbeat or signs of response.

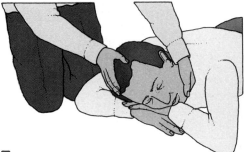

1 With the casualty face down on a hard flat surface, place the arms above the head and place the hands, one over the other, under the head. Turn the head to one side, with the cheek resting on the uppermost hand. Tilt the head back, and extend the jaw so that the casualty's airway is open.

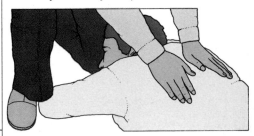

2 Kneel on one knee at the casualty's head with your other foot at the point of the casualty's elbow. Place your hands on the casualty's back on top of the shoulder blades; your thumbs should be along either side of the spine.

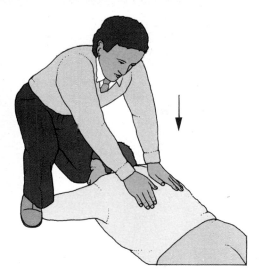

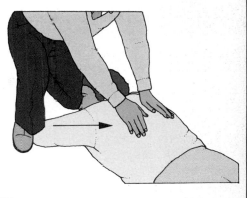

3 Keep your elbows straight and rock forward until your arms are approximately vertical exerting steady pressure for about two seconds. This makes the casualty breathe out.

Do Not apply too much pressure or you may damage lungs and internal organs.

5 Lower the casualty's arms and slide your hands down on to the back again ready to repeat the cycle. Repeat the sequence rhythmically twelve times per minute; each cycle of expansion and compression should last for 5 seconds.

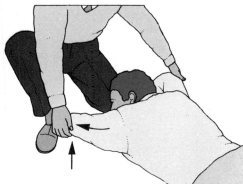

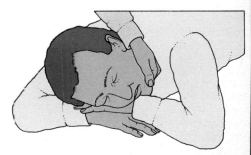

6 After four cycles, check for heartbeat (see p. 17). If it is present continue, but if not, turn the casualty on to the back and perform External Chest Compression and then use the Silvester method of ventilation (see p. 32).

7 As soon as the casualty begins to breathe normally, place in the Recovery Position (see p. 24).

4 Rock backwards, sliding your hands upwards and outwards along the casualty's arms and grasp them just above the elbow. Raise the casualty's arms until resistance and tension are felt at the shoulder, about 3 seconds — this produces inspiration.

Do Not overstretch.

Silvester Method

If a manual method of Artificial Ventilation is needed (for reasons listed on p. 30), and the Holger Nielsen method cannot be used because the casualty is trapped on the back or has to be turned on to the back for External Chest Compression, the Silvester method should be used. However, the Open Airway Position can only be maintained with support under the shoulders.

Method

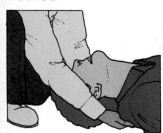 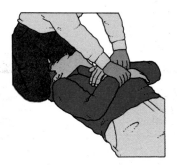 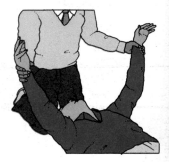

1 Lay the casualty on the back on a firm surface and clear the mouth of any obvious obstructions. Place a folded jacket, or other padding, beneath the shoulders to raise them sufficiently for the head to be tilted back in the Open Airway Position (see p. 15).

2 Kneel at the casualty's head, grasp the wrists, and cross them over on the lower chest, keeping them clear of the abdomen. Rock your body forward and, keeping your back straight, press down firmly on the lower part of the casualty's chest with a steady, even pressure, as with the Holger Nielsen method, for 2 seconds.

3 Release the pressure, rock backwards on your heels and, with a continuous, sweeping movement, draw the casualty's arms upwards and outwards as far as possible, for 3 seconds. Repeat this sequence rhythmically twelve times per minute.

4 After four sequences check for heartbeat. If the heart is beating normally, continue to use the method until natural breathing is restored. If it is absent, give External Chest Compression (see p. 20) and check regularly for response to treatment (see p. 21). If the casualty is not responding, continue resuscitation with fifteen chest compressions to two Silvester ventilations.

5 As soon as the casualty begins to breathe normally, place in the Recovery Position (see p. 24).

Silvester Method with Two First Aiders

If more than one First Aider is present, one should perform the Silvester method and then check for heartbeat, the other should extend the airway by pushing the chin forward, then perform External Chest Compression, if necessary.

ACTION AT AN EMERGENCY

The basic principles of First Aid apply to all injuries or illnesses regardless of severity. Whatever the incident, it is the First Aider's responsibility to act quickly, calmly and correctly in order to preserve life, prevent deterioration in the casualty's condition and promote recovery. These objectives are best achieved by:

● A rapid but calm approach.

● A quick assessment of the situation and the casualty.

● A correct diagnosis of the condition based on the history of the incident, symptoms and signs.

● Immediate and appropriate treatment of any conditions.

● Proper disposal of the casualty according to the injury or condition.

APPROACH

This should be speedy but calm and controlled. Ensure that you are not placing yourself in any danger when approaching the casualty. On arriving at the scene of any incident, state that you are a trained First Aider and, if there are no doctors, nurses or more experienced people present, calmly take charge.

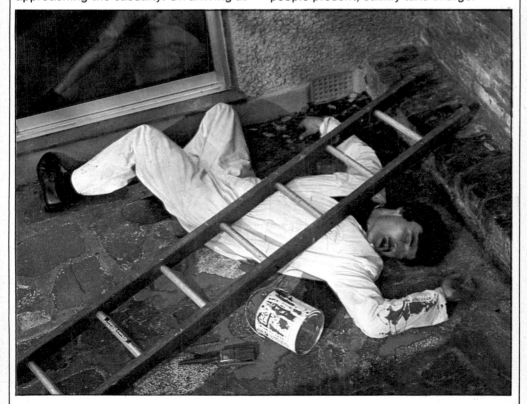

ASSESSING THE SITUATION

As soon as you have taken control, it is crucial that you make an accurate assessment of the situation and decide on the priorities of action.

The conditions which affect these are as follows: Safety, Getting Others to Help, Determining the Priorities of Treatment and Calling for Assistance.

Safety

Minimise the risk of danger to yourself, the casualty and any bystanders, and guard against any further casualties arising. In the case of:
● **Road Accidents** Instruct a bystander to control the traffic, keeping it well away from yourself and the casualty. Watch out for fire risks, especially from petrol spillage and switch off the ignition of the vehicles concerned. (See *Procedure at Major Incidents* p. 168).
● **Gas and poisonous fumes** If possible, cut off the source.
● **Electrical contact** Break the contact, if possible, and take the necessary precautions against further contact.
● **Fire and collapsing buildings** Move the casualty to safety immediately.

Getting Others to Help You

Some bystanders can be extremely useful and may be able to assist with treatment, for example, controlling severe bleeding or supporting a badly injured limb. Other bystanders may become nuisances so you must keep them occupied to prevent them interfering with your work. They can be asked to control traffic or crowds, or be sent to telephone for assistance (see p. 35). However, when sending bystanders to the telephone make sure that they understand the message that is to be sent. If possible, ask them to write it down but, in any case, ask them to repeat the message to you before actually sending it. Always make sure that they report back to you afterwards.

Determining the Priorities of Treatment

In order to determine the condition of a casualty, perform the following checks immediately.

Airway and breathing
Quickly check that the airway is open and that the casualty is breathing. If not, commence Artificial Ventilation immediately (see p. 18).

Bleeding
Check the casualty for any severe bleeding and control it (see p. 28).

Unconsciousness
Place an unconscious casualty, or one whose breathing is noisy, in the Recovery Position (see p. 24) and establish the level of responsiveness (see p. 98). If

there is any possibility of spinal injury *do not* move the casualty (see p. 114), unless difficulty in breathing makes it essential.

Shock

Keep the casualty warm, quiet and lying down until skilled help arrives (see p. 90).

Other Needs

Unless there is immediate danger to life from the surroundings treat all fractures and large wounds before moving a casualty. If the casualty is in danger, temporarily immobilise the injured part before moving.

Calling for Assistance

Once you decide that assistance is required, and this may include ambulance, police, fire brigade, gas or electricity boards, send for it immediately. Go to the nearest telephone, or send a bystander, dial 999 and state the service required, normally ambulance.

Whether you are giving the message yourself or instructing someone to do so make sure that the following information is passed on:

1 Your telephone number (if for any reason you are cut off the officer will then be able to contact you).

2 The exact location of the incident; if you can, point out nearby road junctions or other landmarks.

3 An indication of the type and seriousness of the incident, for example, "Road traffic accident, two cars involved, three people trapped".

4 The number, sex and approximate age of the casualties involved and, if possible, the nature of their injuries.

5 Request special aid if you suspect a heart attack or childbirth.

NB Each control officer has direct access to the other emergency switchboards and will pass on any messages, if necessary.

Do Not replace the receiver before the control officer does so.

Multiple Casualties and Injuries

Where there is more than one casualty, you must decide by rapid assessment which one should receive priority of treatment. You should open the airway of any casualty whose breathing has stopped or is failing and, if necessary, start Artificial Ventilation (see p. 18). Any unconscious casualty should be placed in the Recovery Position immediately (see p. 24), especially if you are working alone. Temporary control of continuous severe bleeding should be effected with the assistance of the casualty or a bystander. Remember that the noisiest casualty is rarely the most severely injured.

It should also be remembered that in First Aid common sense is almost as important as the actual knowledge of the subject. In real life it will be found that serious accidents rarely produce only a single injury. Frequently two or more injuries occur so that the correct treatment of one may interfere with the correct treatment of the other. In such circumstances, you must decide which injury is the more serious and treat that one in the correct way. You should then deal with the second injury as correctly as possible under the conflicting circumstances.

DIAGNOSIS

Having dealt with the priorities (see p. 34), you should then attempt a fuller diagnosis. This takes account of the casualty's *history* (and that of the incident), the *symptoms, signs* and *levels of responsiveness*.

HISTORY

This is the full story of how the incident occurred or the illness began, and should be taken directly from the casualty and a responsible bystander wherever possible. For example, a casualty may only say "I slipped and fell down" whereas a witness may say "I saw the old man fall and his head hit the wall". Pay full attention to the story which may provide clues to the likely injuries and especially if you suspect an existing illness such as diabetes or heart disease. Make a note of details of past similar occurrences and treatments for the examining doctor's benefit later.

Never hurry the casualty and remember to pass on all the information when skilled help arrives.

SYMPTOMS

These are sensations that the casualty feels and describes to you — the most useful of these is pain.

If the casualty is *conscious*, ask if there is any pain and, if so, where. Examine that part first, then run through the various sites at which pain is felt. Remember, however, that a severe pain in one area may mask a more serious injury, which produces less pain, in another. Other useful symptoms the casualty may disclose are nausea, giddiness, feelings of heat and cold, or loss of muscular control or sensation. All symptoms should then be investigated and confirmed by a physical examination for signs of abnormality, such as injury or illness.

If the casualty is *unconscious*, or unreliable because dazed or in shock, then diagnosis cannot be based on symptoms but has to be based on information from bystanders and *signs*.

SIGNS

These are details ascertained by you using your senses — sight, touch, hearing and smell. These may be: signs of injury such as bleeding, swelling, deformity or signs of illness such as a raised temperature and/or a rapid or an irregular pulse.

All these signs may be immediately obvious, noticed incidentally or deliberately discovered by *examination*.

Examination

A general examination should be carried out quickly to discern any imminent threats to life whether the casualty is conscious or unconscious. Move the casualty as little as possible: begin your examination at the casualty's head and work methodically towards the feet. Remember to look, feel, listen and smell and always compare one side of the body with the other.

If at any stage during the examination the casualty's breathing becomes difficult, place the casualty in the Recovery Position (see p. 24).

HEAD

Mouth Re-check *breathing*, noting the rate, depth, and nature (whether easy or difficult, noisy or quiet); note also any *odour*. Check the inside of the mouth quickly to ensure there is no foreign matter in it, such as vomit, blood, food, loose teeth, that might cause choking. Examine the *lips* for any signs of burning or discoloration that might indicate corrosive poisoning. Look inside the lips for any trace of blueness which might indicate asphyxia. Check the *teeth* to make sure that any recently dislodged teeth have not fallen down into the back of the throat. Make sure that dentures are firm-fitting (essential for resuscitation); if they are not they should be removed.

Nose Check for signs of blood, clear fluid or a mixture of both which might come from inside the skull.

Eyes Examine both together noting the resistance of the eyelashes to touch. Compare the pupils (the black circular centres) and note whether they are equal in size. The white orb of the eye should be examined for bloodshot appearance.

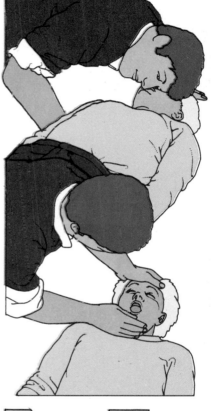

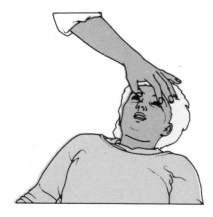

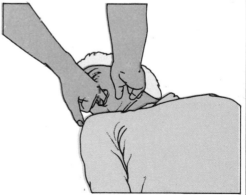

Face Look at the *colour*, it may be pale or flushed, or even bluish if breathing is affected. At the same time, feel the *temperature* of the face to check whether it is particularly hot or cold and note the state of the *skin* – whether it is dry or clammy or even sweating profusely.

Ears These should be checked for foreign bodies and traces of blood and/or clear cerebro-spinal fluid that might indicate skull fracture. Speak into the casualty's ears to test hearing.

Skull Gently run the hands over the scalp searching for bleeding, swelling or indentation that might indicate a fracture.

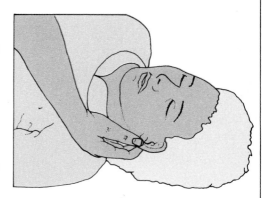

NECK

Loosen clothing around the neck. Run the fingers over the *spine* from the base of the skull down to as far as you can reach between the shoulders, checking for any irregularity of the *vertebrae* that might indicate a fracture. Check round the neck, to see whether any warning *medallion* is being worn. Check the *carotid pulse*, and note its rate, strength, and rhythm (see p. 89). If the casualty is unconscious and the neck is not damaged, place the head in the Open Airway Position (see p. 15).

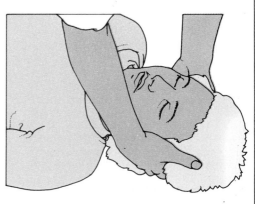

SPINE

Pass your hand gently under the hollow of the back and, without moving the casualty or removing any clothing, feel along the spine as high and as low as you can looking for irregularity of the vertebrae or swelling.

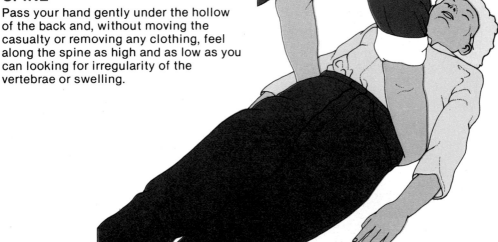

TRUNK

Check the *chest* for evenness of rib movement on breathing and examine for any wounds that might be "sucking" air. Check the *ribs* for irregularity or depression that might indicate a fracture and also feel along the line of the *breastbone*.

Check both *collar-bones* for irregularity and the *shoulders* for signs of deformity. Carefully feel either side of the *pelvis* looking for signs of fracture and note any indication of *incontinence*.

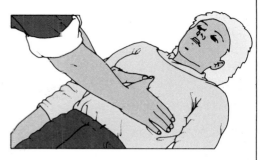

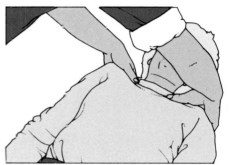

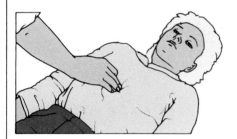

ARMS

The *upper-arm bones*, then the bones in the *forearm*, *wrists*, *hands* and *fingers* should be thoroughly examined. Check carefully for any deformity and swelling which might indicate fractures. The forearms should be checked to see if a casualty is wearing a medical warning bracelet and for injection marks.

LEGS

Check the *hips*, *thighs*, *knee-caps*, both bones of the *lower legs*, the *ankles*, *feet*, and *toes* in the same way as the arms. **NB** Use two hands so that both sides of the body can be examined and compared at the same time.

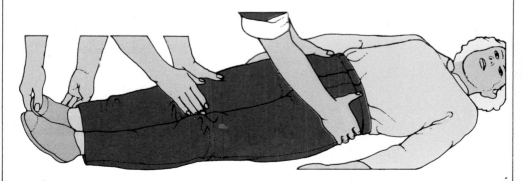

Levels of Responsiveness

There are various stages through which a casualty may pass during progression from consciousness to unconsciousness. These are dealt with in detail on p. 98 but, basically, if the casualty responds well to stimuli then unconsciousness is only light (as in a faint, for example). But if the level of responsiveness is *low* then the casualty is more deeply unconscious. If the response is totally *absent* then the casualty is in a potentially dangerous state.

Every 10 minutes you should re-check and note the casualty's response to the stimuli of *noise* (speak loudly into the ear), *touch* (try to arouse by shaking shoulders gently), *pain* (watch the face while you pinch the skin on hand or ankle) and *reflex action* of the eyelids (touch the eyelashes). In addition, a similar check should be kept on the casualty's breathing (see p. 14), pulse (see p. 89) and temperature, and the findings should be recorded.

Aids to Diagnosis

Your diagnosis is based on information from various sources. By taking the history of the incident, asking the casualty for symptoms and examining the casualty for signs, it should be possible to make an accurate diagnosis. The following chart is a summary of how to achieve this.

HISTORY obtained from surroundings, casualty and bystanders

SYMPTOMS
These are the sensations experienced by the casualty obtained by asking tactful questions.

Pain
Tenderness
Loss of normal movement
Loss of sensation
Cold
Heat
Thirst
Nausea
Weakness
Dizziness
Faintness
Temporary loss of
    consciousness
Loss of memory

SIGNS
Noted by the First Aider's senses

Sight	**Touch**	**Smell**	**Hearing**
Respiration	Dampness	Breath	Breathing
Bleeding	(bleeding,	Burning	Groans
(type and	inconti-	Gas	
volume)	nence)	Alcohol	
Wounds	Temperature		
Foreign	Pulse		
bodies	Swelling		
Colour of	Deformity		
face	Irregularity		
Swelling	Tenderness		
Deformity			
Bruising			
Reflexes			
Responses			
to touch			
and sound			
Incontinence			
Vomit			
Containers			

External Clues

If a casualty is unconscious, the *pockets*, *handbag* or *briefcase*, may have to be checked for possible clues. These may be *appointment cards* for hospital/clinic or *information cards* that might show that the casualty is on steroids or insulin or is liable to epileptic fits. Any lumps of sugar or glucose present might indicate that the casualty is a diabetic. If possible, check this in the presence of a witness.

There are a number of *medical warning items* which can be worn by persons with

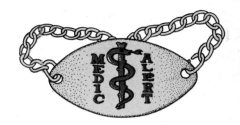

a medical condition. They may take the form of an inscribed medallion or bracelet ("Medic-alert", for example), a locket for wrist or neck or a capsule on a neck chain or key-ring containing a strip of paper describing the condition.

TREATMENT

You should carry out the appropriate treatment for each condition found, gently and quickly. It is most important that you reassure and encourage the casualty constantly. Work calmly and efficiently, pay attention to any remarks or requests that the casualty makes and do not pester with questions. This is annoying for the casualty and is a sign of nervousness on your part. After giving the necessary treatment, place the casualty in the appropriate position and keep a watchful eye until help arrives.

Bear in mind your aim is to preserve life, prevent the condition worsening and promote recovery.

To prevent the condition worsening:
● Dress wounds.
● Immobilise any large wounds and fractures.
● Place the casualty in the most comfortable position consistent with the requirements of treatment.

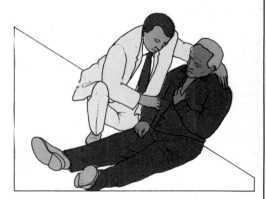

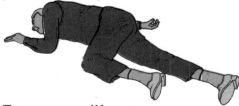

To preserve life:
● Maintain an open airway by positioning the casualty correctly.
● Begin resuscitation if the casualty is not breathing and the heart is not beating and continue treatment until skilled medical aid is available.
● Control bleeding.

To promote recovery:
● Relieve the casualty of anxiety and encourage confidence.
● Attempt to relieve the casualty of pain and discomfort.
● Handle the casualty gently.
● Protect the casualty from the cold and wet.

DISPOSAL OF THE CASUALTY

After you have carried out your treatment the casualty should normally receive attention from a qualified person (doctor or nurse) without undue delay. Depending on the severity of the condition and the availability of skilled help you should:

1 Arrange transport to hospital by ambulance (or by car for minor injuries and arm fractures).

2 Hand over the casualty to the care of a doctor or nurse at the scene.

3 Take the casualty to a nearby house or shelter to await the arrival of the ambulance or doctor.

4 Allow the casualty to go home and advise to seek medical advice, if necessary.

Never send anyone home who has been unconscious, even for a short time, or who is in shock; seek medical aid.

REPORTING ON THE CASUALTY

The casualty should always be accompanied by a brief written report when he or she leaves your care. If necessary, you should accompany the casualty yourself and make a personal report.

The need to supply complete information cannot be emphasised enough, and it should include the following:
● History of the accident or illness.
● Brief description of injury.
● The level of responsiveness and any changes.
● Any other associated injuries.
● The pulse and any changes.
● The skin colour and any changes.
● Blood loss sustained.
● Any unusual behaviour by the casualty.
● Any treatment given and when.

You should also send a tactful message to the casualty's home stating what has happened and where the casualty has been taken if this has not already been done by the police or other authority attending the incident.

Property
Take care of any property belonging to the casualty and hand it over to the police or ambulance personnel.

DEALING WITH CLOTHES AND HELMETS

Sometimes it is necessary to remove clothing in order to expose injuries, make an accurate diagnosis or conduct a proper treatment. This should be done with the minimum of disturbance to the casualty and clothing and only remove as much as is actually necessary. Clothing should not be damaged unnecessarily. If very tight underclothing, such as a girdle, has to be cut, do this along the seams, if it is possible.

If you need to remove the casualty's clothing ensure that sufficient privacy is maintained.

Removing Protective Helmets

Whether or not you remove a protective helmet, such as a motor-cycle crash-helmet, depends on the situation and condition of the casualty. It is best left on and should only be removed if the casualty's condition warrants it. If possible, the helmet should be removed by the casualty. A full-face helmet that encloses the head and face should *only* be removed if it obstructs breathing, if the casualty is vomiting or if there are severe head injuries. In most cases, however, the removal of a helmet will depend entirely on the injuries and your ability to remove it.

To remove a helmet that covers the head only, unfasten or cut through the chinstrap, if necessary. Take pressure off the head by forcing the sides apart, then lift the helmet upwards and backwards.

A full-face helmet needs two persons to remove it safely, one to support the casualty's head and neck, while the other lifts the helmet. First, tilt the helmet back and lift until it is clear of the chin; second, tilt it forward to pass over the base of the skull, then lift it straight off.

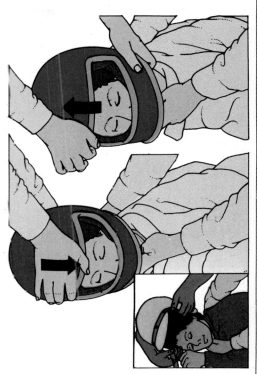

Removing Clothing

REMOVING A COAT OR JACKET

1 Raise the casualty and slip the garment over the shoulders. Bend the arm on the sound side and remove the coat from that side first. Then, slip the injured arm out of its sleeve, keeping the arm straight if possible.

2 If necessary, slit up the seam on the injured side.

REMOVING A SHIRT OR VEST

Remove as for a coat. If necessary, slit it down the front or side.

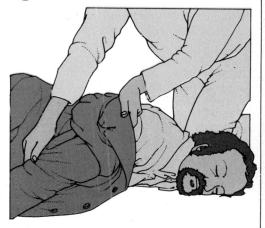

REMOVING TROUSERS

1 Pull them down from the waist to reveal the thigh or raise the trouser leg to expose the calf and knee.

2 If necessary, slit up the inside seam.

REMOVING BOOTS OR SHOES

1 Support the ankle, undo or cut any laces and carefully remove the shoe.

2 If the casualty is wearing long boots, that will not unfasten, carefully slit them down the back seam with a knife.

REMOVING SOCKS

1 If these are difficult to remove, insert your first two fingers between the sock and the leg.

2 Raise the sock and cut it between your fingers.

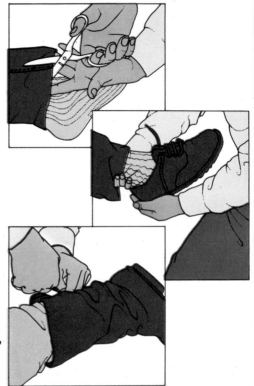

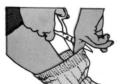

SUMMARY

- Ensure that there is no further danger to the casualty or yourself.
- Act quickly, quietly and methodically, giving priority to the urgent conditions.
- If breathing has stopped, or is failing, open the airway and, if necessary, start Artificial Ventilation.
- Control bleeding.
- Determine the level of responsiveness.
- Reassure the casualty and those around as necessary, so as to lessen any anxiety.
- Guard against shock.
- Position the casualty correctly and comfortably but do not move more than is absolutely necessary.

- Consider the possibility of internal bleeding and poisoning.
- Treat large wounds and fractures before moving the casualty.
- If necessary, arrange without delay for the conveyance of the casualty to a hospital or to the care of a doctor.
- Watch and record any changes.
- Do not attempt too much.
- Do not allow people to crowd round; this hinders First Aid and may cause the casualty anxiety or embarrassment.
- Do not remove clothing unnecessarily.
- Do not give anything by mouth to a casualty who is unconscious, who has a suspected internal injury or who may shortly need an anaesthetic.

ASPHYXIA

This is a potentially fatal condition which occurs if there is not enough oxygen available to the tissues of the body. Such lack may be due to an insufficient amount of oxygen in the air breathed in or any interference with, or injury to, the respiratory system. Without an adequate supply of oxygen, the tissues deteriorate very rapidly: vital nerve cells in the brain can die after only three minutes without oxygen.

There are many conditions which can result in asphyxia some of which are listed below.

Those conditions affecting the airway and lungs include:
● *Obstructed airway* due to the tongue falling into the back of the throat in an unconscious casualty; food, vomit or other foreign body present in the airway; or swelling of the tissues in the throat resulting from scalds, stings or infection.
● *Suffocation* by pillows or plastic bags.
● *Fluid in the air passages.*
● *Compression of the windpipe* by hanging or strangulation.
● *Compression of the chest* caused by a fall of earth or sand, being crushed against a wall or barrier or pressure from a crowd.
● *Injury to the lungs.*
● *Injury to the chest wall*, for example, a stove-in-chest.
● *Fits* preventing adequate breathing.

Those conditions affecting the brain or nerves which control respiration include:
● *Electrical injury.*
● *Poisoning.*
● *Paralysis* caused by a stroke or injury to the spinal cord.

Those conditions affecting the amount of oxygen in the blood include:
● *Air containing insufficient oxygen* such as may be found in gas or smoke-filled buildings or shafts and tunnels.

● *Change in atmospheric pressure* at high altitudes, in depressurized aircraft or when deep sea diving.

Those conditions preventing the use of oxygen in the body include:
● *Carbon-monoxide poisoning.*
● *Cyanide poisoning.*

General Symptoms and Signs
● Difficulty in breathing: the rate and depth of breathing increases.
● Breathing may become noisy with snoring or gurgling.
● Possible frothing at the mouth.
● Blueness of lips and fingernails (cyanosis).
● Confusion.
● Possible unconsciousness.
● Breathing may stop.

Aim
Maintain or restore the casualty's breathing by quickly removing the cause of the asphyxia from the casualty or the casualty from the cause. If necessary, begin Artificial Ventilation (see p. 18) and seek medical aid.

General Treatment
1 Remove the cause of asphyxia and open the airway (see p. 15).

2 If the casualty is not breathing, begin Artificial Ventilation immediately (see p. 18–21).

3 When breathing and pulse return place the casualty in the Recovery Position (see p. 24).

4 Check breathing rate (see p. 12), pulse (see p. 89) and levels of responsiveness (see p. 98) at 10-minute intervals.

5 Seek medical aid as soon as possible.

Suffocation

This results when air is prevented from reaching the air passages by an external obstruction such as a plastic bag, soft pillow or a fall of sand. Suffocation also results from being in a confined space when all the available oxygen has been used up, such as being accidentally shut in an abandoned refrigerator. (For suffocation by smoke, see p. 49.)

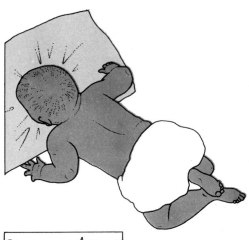

Symptoms and Signs
● General symptoms and signs of asphyxia.
● Obvious air-tight seal over the mouth and nose or presence of "stale" air in a confined space.

Aim
Restore supply of air to the casualty. Resuscitate, if necessary and seek medical aid.

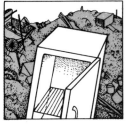

A baby may be suffocated through lying face-down on a pillow. However, being locked in an abandoned refrigerator can also result in suffocation

Treatment

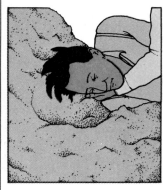

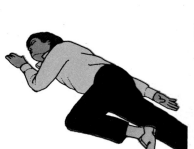

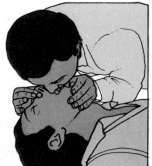

1 Immediately remove any obstruction or remove the casualty to fresh air.

2 If the casualty is conscious and breathing normally, reassure and observe.

3 If the casualty is unconscious but breathing normally, place in the Recovery Position (see p. 24).

4 If breathing is difficult or has stopped, begin Artificial Ventilation immediately (see p. 18).

5 Seek medical aid. If in doubt about the casualty's condition, arrange removal to hospital.

Hanging, Strangling and Throttling

Pressure on the outside of the neck by hanging, strangling or throttling, squeezes the airway shut and blocks off the flow of air to the lungs. *Hanging* involves suspension of the body by the neck from a noose. *Strangling* involves cutting off the air supply by a tight constriction around the neck. *Throttling* involves cutting off the air supply to the neck by intentional squeezing of a person's throat, as in an assault. The first two conditions may occur accidentally. For example, a tie may become caught in machinery.

Aim

Remove the cause of the constriction immediately even if there are no signs of life and, if necessary, commence resuscitation. Arrange removal to hospital.

NB Seek medical aid even if recovery seems complete.

Treatment

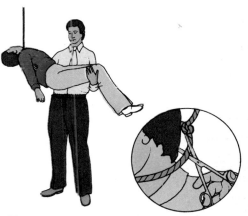

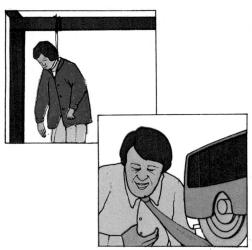

Symptoms and Signs
● General symptoms and signs of asphyxia.
● Congestion of the face and neck with the veins becoming prominent.
● Constriction may still be visible around neck (e.g., a scarf), or it may be hidden in the folds of the skin (e.g., wire).
● There may be marks round the throat or neck where a constriction has been removed.
● Body may still be suspended.

1 Remove the constriction from around the neck immediately, supporting the weight of the body if it is hanging. Take care to cut *below* the knot if any (a knot is difficult to cut and it may be useful evidence).

2 If the casualty is unconscious but breathing normally, place in the Recovery Position (see p. 24).

3 If breathing is difficult or has stopped, begin Artificial Ventilation immediately (see p. 18).

4 Remove to hospital.

Drowning

Drowning causes asphyxia by water entering the lungs or by causing the throat to go into spasm so constricting the air passage (dry drowning). Only small amounts of water can enter the lungs, however, no time should be wasted in trying to remove any water from the casualty's lungs.

Congestion of the lungs can occur very quickly, but it may be several hours before it is apparent. So, all casualties rescued from drowning should be sent to hospital.

If a casualty has been immersed in cold water for a long period there is also a danger of hypothermia (see p. 145),

so it is important that the casualty is kept warm.

Symptoms and Signs
● General symptoms and signs of asphyxia.
● Froth around the casualty's lips, mouth and nostrils.

Aim
Get air into the casualty's lungs as fast as possible, in the water, if necessary. Continue Artificial Ventilation as soon as you can get the casualty on to a firm surface such as the shore or a boat. Arrange removal to hospital.

Treatment

1 Quickly remove any obstructions such as seaweed from the casualty's mouth and begin Artificial Ventilation immediately (see p. 18). If the casualty is still in the water, it may be possible to begin ventilation there.

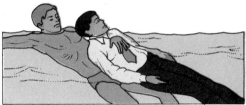

If *in deeper water* give the occasional breath of air while towing the casualty ashore.

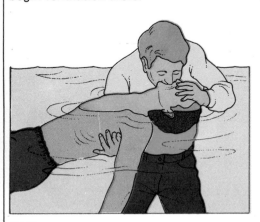

If *within your depth* use one arm to support the casualty's body and use the other hand to support the head and seal the nose while you perform Mouth-to-Mouth Ventilation.

2 When you can place casualty on a firm surface, check breathing (see p. 14) and heartbeat (see p. 17) and continue resuscitation if necessary (pp. 18–21).

3 As soon as the casualty begins breathing normally place in the Recovery Position (see p. 24).

4 Keep the casualty warm. If possible, remove wet clothing and dry off the casualty. Cover with spare clothes and/or towels and, if necessary, treat for Hypothermia (see p. 146).

5 Remove to hospital: transport as a stretcher case maintaining the treatment position.

Smoke Inhalation

A fire uses up oxygen in the atmosphere so the oxygen level in a burning room is low and asphyxia may result. Moreover, smoke may irritate the throat which can go into spasm and close the airway. In addition, the plastic coverings and foam padding of modern upholstery often give off highly toxic fumes when burning which can be fatal.

Symptoms and Signs
● General symptoms and signs of asphyxia.
● Casualty may be scorched or burned.
● Symptoms and signs of shock due to burns (see p. 90).

Aim
Call the emergency services immediately. Only attempt to remove the casualty from the fire and smoke if you can be sure there are *no* toxic fumes present (see *Entering a Gas or Smoke-Filled Room* p. 171). Otherwise, try to extinguish the fire and once the casualty is clear resuscitate if necessary.

Treatment

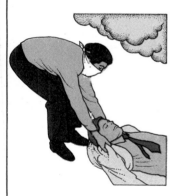
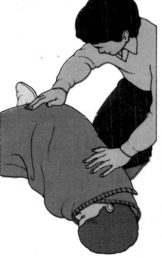
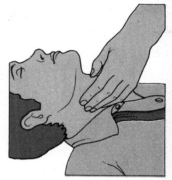

1 Remove the casualty to safety (see p. 171).

2 Extinguish any clothing that is on fire or smouldering (see p. 136).

3 If the casualty is unconscious but breathing normally, place casualty in the Recovery Position (see p. 24).

4 If breathing is difficult or has stopped, begin Artificial Ventilation immediately (see p. 18).

5 Treat any burns (see Burns and Scalds pp. 137–9).

6 Remove to hospital.

Carbon-Monoxide Poisoning

Carbon monoxide is a colourless, odourless gas. Its fumes are dangerous because carbon monoxide replaces the oxygen already present in the blood. It is more readily absorbed by the blood than oxygen and a casualty may require prolonged Artificial Ventilation to clear it completely.

The most common sources of carbon monoxide are fumes from partially burnt fuels and petrol engine exhausts. Danger arises if an exhaust system is defective or if an engine is left running in an enclosed space.

Only enter a gas-filled room to rescue a casualty if you are not in any danger and if you can get out again easily. Make sure you have back-up help so you can get out quickly (see p. 171).

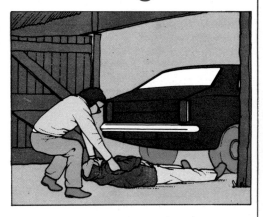

Symptoms and Signs
● General symptoms and signs of asphyxia.
● Casualty may complain of a headache.
● Colour may be normal but will deepen to cherry-pink as the level of carbon monoxide in the blood rises.
● Casualty may be confused and unco-operative.
● Breathing is difficult or may have stopped.
● Unconsciousness may develop.

Aim
Cut off source of gas and/or attempt to remove the casualty from the supply if you are not in any danger. Resuscitate as soon as possible if necessary. Arrange removal to hospital.

Treatment

1 Open any doors and drag the casualty to safety if possible (see p. 171).

2 If casualty is unconscious but breathing normally, place in the Recovery Position (see p. 24).

3 If breathing is difficult or has stopped, begin Artificial Ventilation immediately (see p. 18).

4 Check breathing rate (see p. 12), pulse (see p. 89) and levels of responsiveness (see p. 98) at 10-minute intervals.

5 Remove to hospital.

NB There are many other gases which are dangerous because although they are not toxic, they displace oxygen. *Carbon dioxide* is produced by the incomplete combustion of any fuel and may be found in sewers and similar enclosed spaces. *Butane* and *propane* are used at home and in industry for heating, lighting or refrigerating, and can leak from faulty connections.

Choking

This normally occurs when the airway is partially or totally obstructed by a large, swallowed object or when something goes down the windpipe rather than down the food passage (see p. 11). However, choking can also be caused by muscular spasm. Adults may choke on pieces of food which have been inadequately chewed and hurriedly swallowed; children are at risk because they like putting objects inside their mouths.

. It is imperative that any obstruction be removed as soon as possible. Encourage a conscious choking casualty to cough the obstruction out. If this does not work, first attempt to dislodge it by using gravity and a "jolting" effect (back slapping). Then, and *only* if this fails, should you try to force the remaining air out of the lungs by an abdominal thrust.

Both these techniques can be used by any First Aider on any casualty (infant, child or adult) in any position (sitting, standing or lying down). Both back slaps and abdominal thrusts are administered up to four times in a sequence but if the technique is successful, the full series does not have to be completed.

Always treat a casualty in the position found. If standing or sitting, treat as over; if the casualty is lying down or if you are smaller than the casualty, treat as described for an unconscious casualty.

If the casualty becomes unconscious, you will have to perform Artificial Ventilation in order to try to blow air past the obstruction and into the lungs (see p. 18); in an unconscious casualty, the throat may relax sufficiently to allow air to pass the obstruction.

Symptoms and Signs

● General symptoms and signs of asphyxia.
● Casualty will be unable to speak or breathe and may be gripping the throat.
● Congestion of the face and neck with the veins becoming prominent; blueness of the lips and mouth.
● Possible unconsciousness.

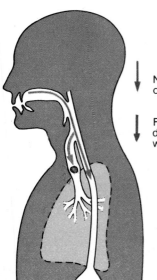

Normal passage of food

Food inhaled down windpipe

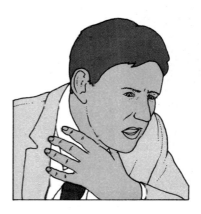

Aim

Try to remove the obstruction; if unsuccessful, begin Artificial Ventilation. If the casualty is unconscious, if choking is prolonged or if recovery is not complete, arrange removal to hospital.

Treatment

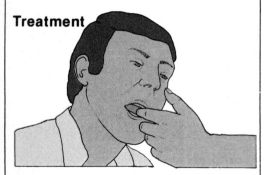

1 Remove any debris or false teeth from the casualty's mouth and encourage the casualty to cough.

2 Help the casualty to bend over with the head lower than the lungs. Slap the casualty smartly between the shoulder-blades with the heel of the hand up to four times; each slap should be hard enough to remove the obstruction by itself.

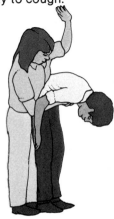

3 Check the mouth to see if the obstruction has been dislodged. If it has not, you may be able to remove it by performing abdominal thrust (see p. 54).

4 Check the mouth again. If the obstruction is visible but not coughed out, hook it out with your fingers.

5 If choking is not relieved, repeat back slaps (up to four times) and abdominal thrusts (up to four times). If casualty becomes unconscious treat as described right.

NB The casualty may begin breathing again at any stage. When this happens advise the casualty to sit quietly and give sips of water as necessary.

FOR THE UNCONSCIOUS CHOKING CASUALTY

1 Turn the casualty on to the back, open the airway (see p. 15) and begin Artificial Ventilation (see p. 18).

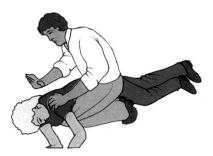

2 If this is not successful, roll the casualty on to the side facing you with the chest against your thigh and the head well back (see p. 24) and perform up to four back slaps as described left.

3 Check the mouth to see if the obstruction has been dislodged. If it has, hook it out with your finger. If it has not, turn the casualty on to the back with the head in the Open Airway Position and perform abdominal thrust (see p. 54).

4 Check the mouth again to see if the obstruction has been dislodged.

5 If choking persists, reposition the casualty's head and attempt Artificial Ventilation (see p. 18). Then repeat steps 1 to 4 as necessary.

6 When the obstruction has been removed and the casualty is breathing normally, place in the Recovery Position (see p. 24) and remove to hospital.

FOR CHILDREN

Many children are comparable in height and build with small adults and can be treated in the same way using slightly less pressure. However, some modifications have to be made if you are treating a small child.

Follow the sequence described for adults but sit in a chair or kneel on one knee and lay the child over your knee, head down. Support the chest with one hand and slap the child smartly between the shoulder-blades up to four times with your other hand. If this does not dislodge the obstruction it may be necessary to perform abdominal thrust (see p. 55).

If the child is or becomes unconscious, place on a firm surface and follow sequence described for unconscious adults.

FOR INFANTS

The order of treatment for infants is the same as for children (see left) but *much* lighter pressure is used and the positions for back slapping and abdominal thrust are different.

Lay the infant's head downwards with the chest and abdomen lying along your forearm and use your arm to support the head and chest. Slap the infant smartly between the shoulders up to four times. If this does not dislodge the obstruction it may be necessary to perform abdominal thrust (see p. 55).

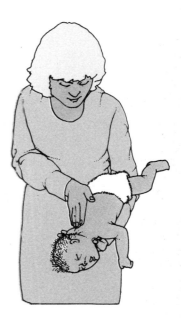

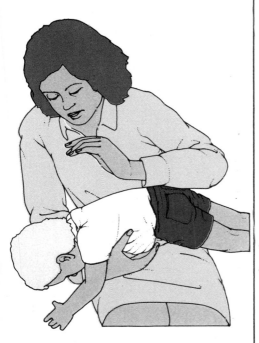

NB Use extreme caution when removing an obstruction from the mouth of an infant. Only put your finger in the mouth if you can see the obstruction and there is no danger of pushing the obstruction further down the throat.

Abdominal Thrust

This is a technique which involves applying a series of thrusts to the upper abdomen in an attempt to force air out of a choking casualty's lungs. However, because there is a possibility that the action required can damage the underlying organs, abdominal thrust must only be used as a last resort after back slapping has failed.

Method

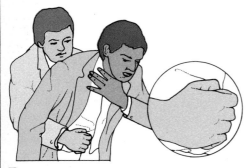

1 Stand or kneel behind the casualty and put one arm around the abdomen. Clench your fist and place it, thumb inwards in the centre of the upper abdomen, between the navel and the breastbone.

2 Grasp your fist with your other hand.

3 Pull both hands towards you with a quick upward and inward thrust from the elbows so that you compress the upper abdomen against the bottom of the lungs. Repeat up to four times as necessary; each thrust must be hard enough to dislodge the obstruction.

FOR THE UNCONSCIOUS CASUALTY

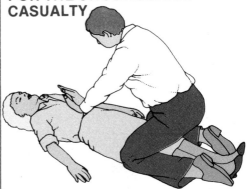

1 Turn the casualty on to the back with the head in the Open Airway Position (see p. 15). Kneel astride the casualty's thighs so that you can apply sufficient pressure at the correct mid-abdominal position. If you cannot straddle the casualty, kneel alongside.

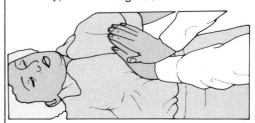

2 Place the heel of one hand in the centre of the casualty's upper abdomen and cover with your other hand keeping fingers clear of the abdomen.

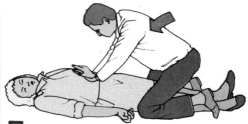

3 With both arms straight, press into the abdomen with a quick inward and forward thrust. Repeat up to four times as necessary; each thrust must be hard enough to dislodge the obstruction.

FOR CHILDREN

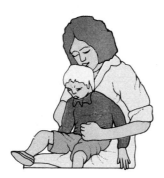

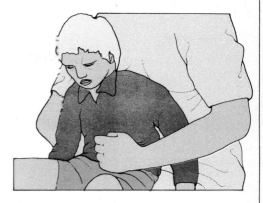

1 Sit the child on your lap or stand the child in front of you and place one arm around the abdomen. Clench your fist and place it thumb inwards in the centre of the upper abdomen, as above. Support the back with your other hand.

2 Press your clenched fist into the abdomen with a quick upward and inward movement using much less pressure than for an adult. Repeat up to four times as necessary; each thrust must be hard enough to dislodge the obstruction by itself.

If the child is unconscious place in the same position as for an unconscious adult. Use the same method but only use one hand and less pressure.

FOR INFANTS

Place the infant on a firm surface with the head in the Open Airway Position (see p. 15). Place the first two fingers of one hand on the upper abdomen, between the navel and the breastbone and press with a quick forward and downward movement. Repeat up to four times as necessary; each thrust must be hard enough to dislodge the obstruction.

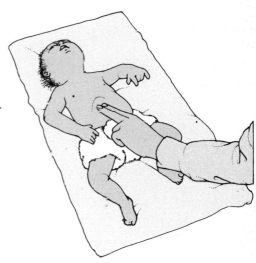

Blast Injuries

Explosions can result from a bomb or if a flame or electrostatic discharge, from a doorbell or telephone for example, is introduced into an area where a combustible gas has been accumulating. The wave of high pressure from the blast may damage the lungs and other organs of the body.

The casualty may also be suffering from extensive burns, fractures, damaged eardrums and other injuries due to flying glass or other debris.

Symptoms and Signs
● General symptoms and signs of asphyxia.
● Frothy, blood-stained spit may be coughed up.
● Casualty may be anxious.
● Probability of multiple injuries.
● Bleeding from the ear if the eardrum is damaged (see p. 74).
● Symptoms and signs of shock (see p. 90).

Aim
Reassure the casualty and treat where found unless the possibility of further explosions exists. Arrange urgent removal to hospital.

Treatment

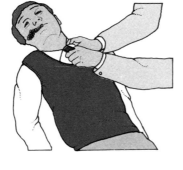

1 Reassure the casualty and move as little as possible until a full examination reveals the extent of the injuries (see *Examination* pp. 36 – 39).

2 If the casualty's general condition and injuries allow, help the casualty into a half-sitting position. Support the head and shoulders.

3 Loosen any constricting clothing around the neck, chest and waist.

4 Control bleeding and treat any wounds (see pp. 64–7) or burns (see pp. 137–9). Immobilise fractures (see pp. 106–127).

5 Check breathing rate (see p. 12), pulse (see p. 89) and levels of responsiveness (see p. 98) at 10-minute intervals.

6 If the casualty becomes unconscious but is breathing normally, place in the Recovery Position (see p. 24).

7 If breathing is difficult or has stopped, begin Artificial Ventilation immediately, (see p. 18).

8 Remove to hospital immediately: transport as a stretcher case maintaining the treatment position.

Stove-in-Chest

Multiple fractures of the chest wall result in the area losing its rigidity and prevent it following the normal movements of the rib cage during breathing (see p. 12). Instead, the fractured ribs are sucked in during breathing-in and pushed out during breathing-out. This is a reversal of the normal movement of the rib cage and the opposite of what is happening on the sound side. This condition is known as *paradoxical breathing* and it may also inhibit the lung action on the uninjured side. In addition to this, the broken bones may damage other internal organs or penetrate the skin causing a "sucking" wound (see p. 80).

Common causes of this type of injury are road traffic accidents in which the driver of a vehicle is thrown against the steering column or the steering column is pushed back into the driver's chest.

The same effect can result if the chest is crushed by heavy objects.

Symptoms and Signs
● General symptoms and signs of asphyxia.
● Casualty finds it difficult and painful to breathe.
● Casualty may be very distressed.
● Unusual movement in the rib cage. Injured part of the chest wall will be seen to have lost its rigidity.
● Possibility of frothy blood-stained spit indicating lung damage (see *Penetrating Wound of the Chest* p. 79).

Aim
Stabilise the chest wall in order to ease breathing. Arrange urgent removal to hospital.

Treatment

1 Support the affected part of the casualty's rib cage with your hand.

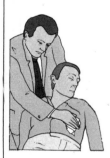

2 Help the casualty into a half-sitting position inclined towards the injured side. Support head and shoulders.

3 If there is a "sucking" wound treat as on p. 81.

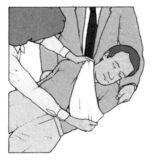

4 Immobilise the chest wall. Place a thick pad of soft material over the injured area and place the arm on the injured side across the pad and support in an Elevation sling (see p. 182). Apply a broad bandage over the sling and right around the body; tie off in front on the uninjured side. If no bandage is available, a scarf or belt may be used.

5 Loosen any constricting clothing around the neck and waist.

6 Check for any signs of other injury.

7 If casualty becomes unconscious, place in the Recovery Position with the sound side uppermost (see p. 24).

8 Remove to hospital immediately: transport as a stretcher case maintaining the treatment position.

Electrical Injuries

The passage of electrical current through the body may result in severe and sometimes fatal injuries. The current can come from a low or high voltage supply or lightning. The electricity can cause quivering of the heart muscle (fibrillation) or it can cause the heart to stop completely which will also result in a cessation of breathing. The casualty may also have severe burns where the electricity enters the body as well as where it leaves the body to "earth". The higher the voltage which passes through the body the more extensive the burns.

Low-voltage appliances and cables in workshops, homes, offices and shops can cause electrical injuries. Most appliances and cables are insulated by non-conducting materials such as plastic or rubber to provide protection from the current. Many injuries result from faulty switches, frayed cables or defects within the appliances themselves. Young children are at risk because they may try to play with switches, wires and plugs.

Water is an excellent conductor of electricity so that handling an otherwise safe appliance with wet hands or when standing on a wet floor, increases the risk of electrical injury.

Lightning is a natural source of electricity which occurs during a thunderstorm. It seeks contact with the ground through the nearest tall feature in the landscape. A person may be hit if in contact with, or standing near, isolated features such as trees, towers or pylons or simply by being the tallest feature in flat area.

The current produced by lightning is of extremely short duration but, whilst it may only stun the casualty, it can also cause instant death; clothing may be set on fire. A casualty should always be removed from a dangerous area as soon as possible.

Whatever the cause of the electrical injury, *never* touch the casualty with bare

BREAKING A LOW-VOLTAGE CURRENT

Break the contact by switching off the current at the mains or meter if it can be quickly reached; if not, remove the plug or wrench the cable free.

If you cannot break the current in this way, stand on some dry insulating material, such as a wooden box, rubber mat or newspaper and, by means of a brush, wooden chair or stool, push the casualty's limbs away from the source.

Alternatively, loop a rope or tights around the casualty's feet or under the arms and pull the casualty away from the source.

NB Avoid using anything metallic or damp or allowing your hands to touch the casualty's flesh. If nothing else is available, grasp the casualty's loose, dry clothing and pull.

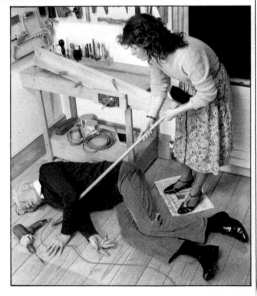

hands until you are sure that there is no further danger to yourself and that the casualty is no longer in contact with the source. In the case of injury from high-voltage electricity do not approach the casualty until you are informed by the police or similar authority that it is safe to do so (see below).

Symptoms and Signs

● General symptoms and signs of asphyxia but casualty's face may be ashen because breathing and heartbeat have stopped simultaneously.

● Deep contact burns may be present at points of entry and exit.

● Symptoms and signs of shock (see p. 90).

Aim

Break the current or remove the casualty from the source if it is safe to do so. Arrange removal to hospital, if necessary.

Treatment

1 If breathing and heartbeat have stopped, begin resuscitation immediately (see p. 18–21).

2 If the casualty is unconscious but breathing normally, place in the Recovery Position (see p. 24).

3 Treat any burns (see pp. 137–9). Examine them carefully; they may be deeper than they appear at first.

4 To minimise shock, treat as on p. 90.

5 Remove to hospital in all cases where a casualty required resuscitation, was unconscious, sustained burns or developed any of the symptoms and signs of shock.

NB Pass on any information you have about duration of electrical contact.

INJURIES FROM HIGH-VOLTAGE ELECTRICITY

Contact with high-voltage currents found in power lines and overhead railway cables is usually immediately fatal. Severe burns always result and the force of sudden muscular spasm caused by the electricity may throw the casualty some distance from the point of contact.

If a casualty remains in contact with, or is still within 18 m (20 yd) of, a high-voltage current, *never attempt to rescue or even approach* until the power has been cut off by the authorities. This is because the electricity may "arc" and jump considerable distances. Insulating material such as dry wood or clothing will not provide any protection.

Make immediate arrangements for the police to be called. Keep any bystanders away from the casualty and only give First Aid when you are officially informed that there is no further danger.

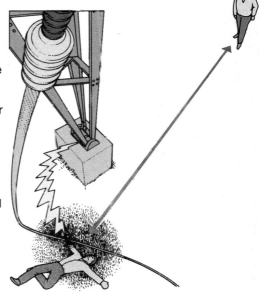

Asthma

Asthma is a distressing condition in which the muscles in the air passages go into spasm. The airway becomes constricted making breathing, particularly breathing out, very difficult. Asthma attacks can be triggered off by nervous tension or an allergy, although in many cases there is no obvious cause. Sudden attacks of difficult breathing sometimes occur at night. Regular asthma sufferers usually carry their own medication in the form of an aerosol to ease breathing in which case they will generally know how to cope with an attack.

Symptoms and Signs
● Casualty may be very anxious and find it difficult to speak.
● Difficulty in breathing, especially breathing out.
● Blueness of the face.

Aim
Reassure and calm the casualty. If possible, provide a source of fresh air and place casualty in a position which will ease breathing. Seek medical aid for prolonged or repeated attacks or if you are in doubt about the casualty's condition.

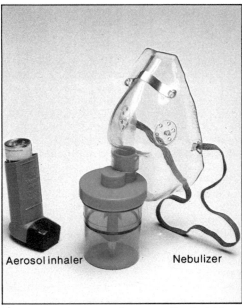

Aerosol inhaler   Nebulizer

Treatment

1 Reassure and calm the casualty.

2 Advise the casualty to sit down leaning slightly forward and rest on a support such as a table. Ensure a good supply of fresh air.

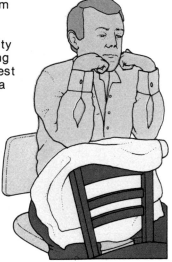

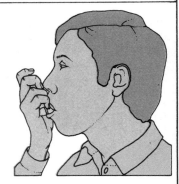

3 If the casualty has medication allow the casualty to take it because it may provide relief.

4 If the symptoms persist or recur seek medical aid.

Winding

A severe blow to or a heavy fall on the upper part of the abdomen (solar plexus) can upset the regularity of breathing.

Symptoms and Signs
- General symptoms and signs of asphyxia, if prolonged.
- Difficulty in breathing-in.
- Casualty may be unable to speak.
- Casualty will be clutching the upper abdomen and is bent double.
- Possible nausea and vomiting.

Aim
Place casualty in a position where breathing is eased. Seek medical aid only if the casualty does not make a full recovery quite quickly.

Treatment
1 Sit the casualty in a relaxed breathing position; if unconscious, place in the Recovery Position (see p. 24).

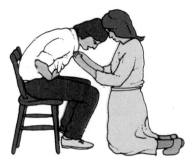

2 Loosen any constricting clothing around the neck, chest and waist.

3 Gently massage the upper abdomen.

Hiccups

Repeated, noisy intakes of air - hiccups - are caused by involuntary contractions of the diaphragm. Hiccuping attacks generally do not last more than a few minutes and are usually only a minor irritation to the sufferer.

Aim
Break up the sequence of these involuntary contractions and seek medical aid if attack is prolonged or severe.

Treatment
1 Ask the casualty to sit quietly and hold the breath or give long drinks.

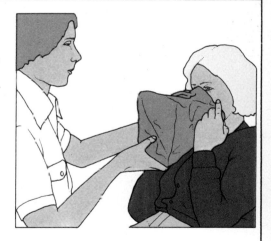

2 If this is unsuccessful, place a *paper*, not plastic, bag over the casualty's mouth and nose, and ask the casualty to breathe in and out.

3 If hiccups persist for more than a few hours, seek medical aid.

WOUNDS AND BLEEDING

To operate efficiently the body has to have enough blood circulating at sufficient pressure to reach all the body's tissues all the time. Severe blood loss interferes with the circulation and this can damage the tissues, especially those of the major organs; this may result in the death of the casualty (see *Dangers of Blood Loss* p. 27).

A wound is an abnormal break in the skin or other tissues which allows blood to escape. External wounds are complicated by the fact that germs (bacteria) can enter the tissues and cause infection.

Types of Wound

Wounds are classified as open or closed. Open wounds allow blood to escape from the body. There are several types: incised wounds, lacerated wounds, puncture wounds, grazes and gunshot wounds.

Closed wounds allow blood to escape from the circulatory system, but not the body. They may be seen as bruises or collections of blood under the skin or there may be no external evidence.

Incised Wound
A knife, razor or sharp edge of paper may cause an incised wound. This type of wound may bleed profusely because cleanly-cut blood vessels do not contract easily.

Lacerated Wound
The skin may be torn irregularly by contact with barbed wire, machinery or the claws of an animal. These wounds tend to bleed less severely than incised wounds because torn blood vessels contract more quickly than cleanly-cut ones; clotting is relatively easy across the jagged edges. These wounds are sometimes contaminated.

Puncture Wound
Nails, needles, garden forks, railings, even teeth, can cause wounds which may result in serious internal injury. If the wound is deep, the risk of infection is high because germs and dirt may have been carried into it.

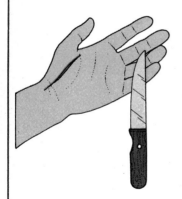
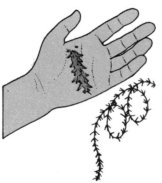
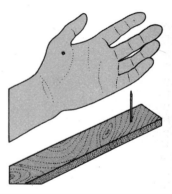

Graze

A graze normally results from a sliding fall. Superficial layers of skin are scraped off leaving a tender, raw area. These wounds often contain dirt or grit which has become embedded during the injury and may easily become infected.

Certain friction burns (see p. 134) where the skin has been broken are treated as grazes.

Gunshot Wound

Gunshot wounds can result in serious internal injury. There will be a wound where a bullet enters the body and often a much larger exit wound. Internal organs, tissues and blood vessels may be damaged during the bullet's passage through the body. In addition to external bleeding, there may be internal bleeding.

Contused Wound

This can be caused by a fall or a blow with a blunt object which splits the skin and bruises the surrounding tissues. In a contused wound the risk of damage to underlying structures (e.g., fracture), should be considered.

With a bruise, damaged blood vessels leak blood into the tissues although the skin remains unbroken (see p. 85).

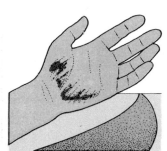

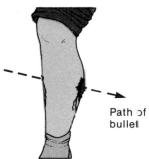

Path of bullet

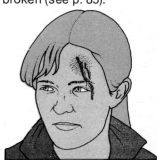

Types of Bleeding

There are three different types of bleeding: arterial, venous and capillary. Each is named after the type of blood vessel damaged (see *Blood and the Circulation*, p. 26). Major arterial bleeding is the most serious and *must* always be treated first (see *Dangers of Blood Loss*, p. 27). Capillary bleeding is always present, however, in some wounds arterial and venous bleeding will also be evident.

Arterial Bleeding

Blood carried in the arteries is normally fully oxygenated and is bright red. It has just come from the heart so it is under pressure and often spurts from a wound in time with the heartbeat.
NB Blood in the artery which takes blood from the heart to the lungs is not fully oxygenated.

Venous Bleeding

Normally darker red because it contains less oxygen, venous blood flows at a lower pressure than arterial blood and will not spurt. It may, however, gush profusely if a major vein is ruptured.

Capillary Bleeding

The capillaries contain both arterial and venous blood and capillary bleeding is the most common type. It is present in any wound and it may be the only type in minor wounds where blood oozes from the wound.

How the Body Responds to Injury

The natural response of the body is to restrict blood flow which minimises blood loss. Almost immediately, the ends of the damaged blood vessels contract to stem the leakage of blood and the blood pressure drops so that less blood is pushed out. If the wound is large, the outer (peripheral) blood vessels which carry blood to the skin and muscles constrict allowing the major blood vessels to carry sufficient blood to the vital organs.

When the blood leaves the damaged vessels it solidifies to form a clot. This clot plugs the blood vessels and seals the wound.

The body then begins to repair the damage. It brings a defence mechanism into play in order to combat local infection (see p. 68). The repair procedures will result initially in a swelling of the tissues because red and white cells and serum which escape from the damaged vessels collect in the area.

Cross-section of Skin Showing Damaged Area

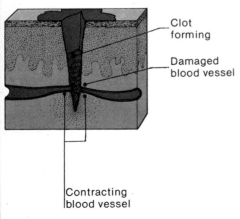

Clot forming

Damaged blood vessel

Contracting blood vessel

Major External Bleeding

This occurs most often after a deep incision or laceration in the skin. It is dramatic and may distract you from the priorities of treatment (see p. 34).

Always remember that if casualty is not breathing, begin Artificial Ventilation immediately (see p. 18); if the casualty is unconscious, maintain an open airway (see p. 14) and then treat the bleeding. Otherwise, treat the casualty in the position which is most effective.

Major bleeding must be treated as soon as possible. In some cases you may find that it is only possible to reduce, not actually stop, the flow of blood but this may be enough to preserve life.

Follow the order of treatment laid out opposite. Apply direct pressure to a wound first and only if this is not possible or effective and you suspect arterial bleeding, apply indirect pressure (see p. 29). Finally, position the casualty to control blood flow.

Symptoms and Signs
● Evidence of major external blood loss.
● Symptoms and signs of shock (see p. 90).
Casualty complains of thirst.
Vision may be blurred and casualty feels faint and giddy.
Face and lips become pale.
Skin feels cold and clammy.
Pulse becomes faster but weaker.
Casualty becomes restless and talkative.
Breathing becomes shallower, sometimes accompanied by yawning and sighing (air hunger).
Possible unconsciousness.

Aim
Control bleeding as soon as possible. Keep the wound clean and dress it to minimise blood loss and prevent infection. Arrange urgent removal to hospital.

Treatment

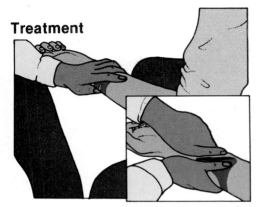

1 Expose the wound and check for the presence of foreign bodies (see p. 66). Apply direct pressure to control bleeding by pressing with fingers or palm of hand (see p. 28). If the wound is large, squeeze the edges together.

2 Lay the casualty down. If the wound is on a limb and you do not suspect a fracture, raise and support it.

3 If the injury is on a limb and direct pressure is ineffective, apply indirect pressure to the main artery which supplies the limb (see p. 29).

Do Not apply indirect pressure for any longer than 15 minutes (see p. 29) nor apply a tourniquet.

4 Place a sterile, unmedicated dressing over the wound, making sure that it extends well beyond the edges of the wound. Press it down firmly and secure with a bandage. Tie bandage firmly enough to control bleeding but not so tight as to cut off circulation (see p. 178). Immobilise the injured part (see *Fractures* pp. 106–127).

If no suitable dressing is available, place a piece of gauze over the wound, cover it with a pad of cotton wool and bandage firmly. An improvised dressing can be made from any suitable material (see p. 175).

5 If bleeding continues, apply further dressings or pads *on top of the original ones* and bandage firmly.

6 To minimise shock, treat as on p. 90.

7 Remove to hospital immediately.

AMPUTATIONS

Recent advances in surgery have made the re-attachment of amputated limbs, fingers and toes possible. The chances of a good result are greater the sooner the casualty and the severed part are removed to hospital. Always place the severed part in a suitable container to protect it. Inform the ambulance service of an amputation injury immediately so that the hospital can prepare for the specialist surgery required.

Aim

Control bleeding and remove casualty to hospital as soon as possible with the severed part.

Treatment

1 Control bleeding using direct pressure, see above; take great care not to damage the stump.

2 Place the severed part in a clean plastic bag to keep it clean and prevent it drying out. If possible, put the bag in a container of ice. However, the bag must be wrapped in suitable material to prevent the severed part touching the ice.

NB Mark the package clearly with the casualty's name and the time the amputation occurred.

3 Remove to hospital immediately.

FOREIGN BODIES

Carefully remove any small, foreign bodies from the surface of a wound if they can be wiped off easily with a swab or rinsed off with cold water.

If the casualty has a large foreign body embedded in the skin, *never* attempt to remove it. It may be plugging the wound therefore restricting bleeding. Moreover, the surrounding tissues may be injured further if it is pulled out.

Treatment

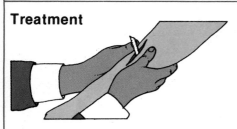

1 To control bleeding, apply direct pressure by squeezing the edges of the wound together alongside the foreign body (see p. 28).

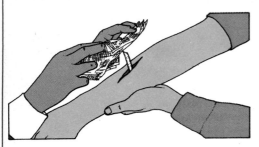

2 Gently place a piece of gauze over and/or around the foreign body.

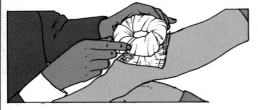

3 Place a ring pad or crescent-shaped pads of cotton wool or similar material around the wound. If possible, build up the padding until it is high enough to prevent pressure on the object.

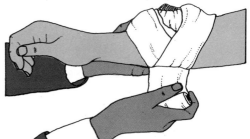

4 Secure with a diagonally applied bandage (see p. 187). Make sure bandage is not over the foreign body.

5 Elevate the injured part and immobilise as far as possible (see *Fractures* pp. 106–127).

6 Remove to hospital immediately maintaining treatment position.

If severe bleeding persists use indirect pressure (see p. 29).

If the casualty is impaled on railings or other spikes, do not attempt to lift off, but make the casualty comfortable by supporting the weight of the limbs and trunk. Call an ambulance immediately asking Control to notify the Fire-brigade because cutting tools may be required (see *Calling for Assistance*, p. 35).

Minor External Bleeding

Many wounds are relatively trivial and involve only slight bleeding. Although blood may ooze from all parts of the wound, it will soon stop of its own accord. A small adhesive dressing is normally all that is necessary, and medical aid need only be sought if there is a serious risk of infection (see p. 72).

Symptoms and Signs
● Pain at the site of the wound.
● Steady trickle of mixed blood.

Aim
Clean and dress the wound as soon as possible to minimise infection.

Treatment

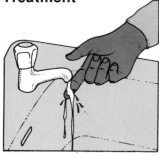

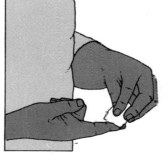

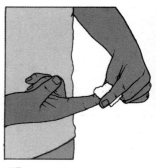

1 If possible wash your hands before dealing with the wound. Then, if the wound is dirty, lightly rinse it with running water, if available, until it is clean.

2 Temporarily protect the wound with a sterile swab. Carefully clean the surrounding skin with water and soap if available. Gently wipe away from the wound using each swab once only and taking care not to wipe off any blood clots. Dab gently to dry.

3 If bleeding persists apply direct pressure (see p. 28).

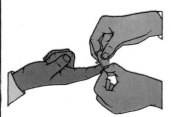

5 Raise and support the injured part unless you suspect an underlying fracture.

6 If in any doubt about the injury, seek medical aid.

If the wound is larger, apply a sterile unmedicated dressing or gauze and clean pad and bandage firmly in position.

4 Dress a small wound with an adhesive dressing (see p. 175).

Infected Wounds

All open wounds will be contaminated by germs which either come from the cause of the injury, from the air or from the First Aider's breath or fingers. Some particles of dirt may be carried away from the damaged tissue by bleeding. Any harmful germs which remain are usually destroyed by the white cells in the blood and the wound then stays clean and healthy (see below).

Normal First Aid treatment for wounds includes prevention of infection. However, any wound which has not begun to heal properly after about 48 hours may be infected because either dirt, dead tissue, foreign bodies and/or bacteria may still be present. If infection develops, it can have serious consequences. It may enter the blood system and subsequently spread to other parts of the body permanently destroying tissue and occasionally leading to death.

Symptoms and Signs

● Increasing pain and soreness in the wound.
● Increased swelling and redness of the wound and surrounding parts with a feeling of heat.
● Pus may ooze from the wound.
● Fever, sweating, thirst, shivering and lethargy if the infection is severe.
● Swelling and tenderness in glands.
● Faint red trails (infected lymph vessels) may be seen on the surface of the inside of the arms or legs leading towards the lymph glands.

Aim

Seek medical aid as soon as possible.

The Lymphatic System

This is a network of hair-like vessels joined up at intervals with small structures called lymphatic nodes (glands) which all help to protect the body against infection. A fluid known as lymph flows from the tissues through these vessels and contains white cells (leucocytes) which may have engulfed germs in the body. As the lymph passes through the lymph glands, it deposits white cells. The lymph glands help trap and dispose of this material and prevent it re-entering the blood stream.

There are three main areas of superficial glands: the neck, armpits, and groin. When these glands are stimulated into action by infection, they become swollen and painful.

The lymph glands
This diagram shows the three main areas of lymph glands in the body.

Treatment

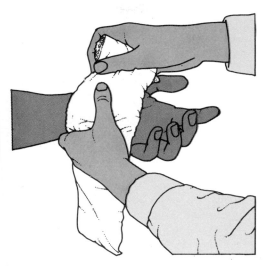

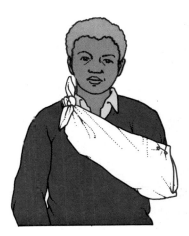

1 Dress wound with prepared sterile unmedicated dressing or similar clean, preferably sterile, material and secure with a bandage.

2 Elevate the injured part and immobilise especially if swollen.

3 Remove to hospital.

TETANUS INFECTION (LOCKJAW)

This particularly dangerous infection results from a toxic substance produced by tetanus germs in a wound spreading into the body's nerves and causing severe muscular spasm, particularly in the jaw, hence the name "Lockjaw". It is a difficult condition to treat which, if it is not treated at an early stage, can lead to the death of a casualty.

Every wound carries the risk of infection. However, the risk of tetanus infection is greater in a dirty wound, especially if it is contaminated by soil from places where animals graze; in deep wounds containing dead tissue; or in wounds where there is a foreign body.

Everyone should be inoculated against tetanus regularly and you should always ask a wounded casualty how recently inoculation was given. Any casualty with a wound who has never had an anti-tetanus injection or who has not kept the protection up-to-date, should be referred to medical aid.

Internal Bleeding

This may occur following an injury such as a fracture or crush injury or because of a medical condition such as a bleeding stomach ulcer. Internal organs, the spleen and liver for example, can be damaged by blows to the body although there may be no external evidence.

Internal bleeding is as serious as external bleeding. Although the blood is not actually lost from the body, it is lost from the circulatory system and the vital organs become starved of oxygen (see *Dangers of Blood Loss* p. 27). Blood collecting internally may also cause problems if it presses on vital structures. For example, blood inside the skull can compress the brain causing loss of consciousness; bleeding inside the chest may prevent the lungs expanding.

Blood from internal injuries may collect in one of the body's cavities and remain concealed. Alternatively, it may be revealed by a flow of blood from one or more of the various openings (orifices) of the body such as the mouth or rectum (see chart overleaf) or by the appearance of discoloration and bruising.

Always suspect internal bleeding after a violent injury, if there are symptoms and signs of shock without any visible blood loss or if there is any "patterned" bruising corresponding to the seams and/or texture of the casualty's clothing.

Symptoms and Signs
These will vary according to the amount and the rate at which blood is lost.
● History of sufficient injury to cause internal bleeding.
● History of a medical condition which may cause internal bleeding (e.g., ulcer).
● Pain and tenderness around the affected area; swelling and tension may be felt.
● Symptoms and signs of shock (see p. 90).
Breathing becomes shallow, sometimes accompanied by yawning and sighing (air hunger).
Casualty becomes restless and talkative.
Casualty complains of thirst.
● Blood may appear from one of the body's orifices (see overleaf).

Aim
Arrange removal to hospital immediately because it is not usually possible to control internal bleeding using First Aid.

Treatment

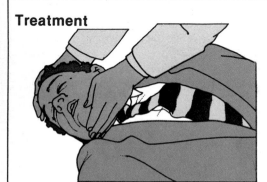

1 Lay the casualty down with the head low and to one side to ensure a good blood supply to the brain. Advise the casualty not to move.

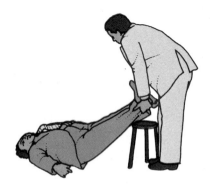

2 If the casualty's injuries allow, raise the legs to aid the return of blood flow to the vital organs.

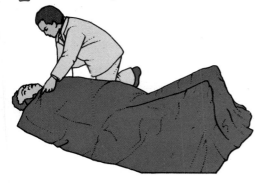

3 Loosen any constricting clothing around the neck, chest and waist.

4 Reassure the casualty and explain the necessity to relax.

5 To minimise shock, treat as on p. 90.

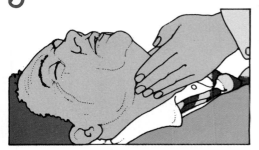

6 Check breathing rate (see p. 12), pulse (see p. 89), and levels of responsiveness (see p. 98) at 10-minute intervals. Record these for the Doctor.

7 Examine the casualty for other injuries (see pp. 36 – 39) and treat as necessary.

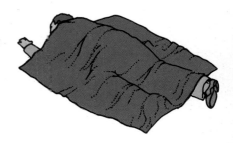

8 If the casualty becomes unconscious but is breathing normally place in the Recovery Position (see p. 24).

9 If breathing and heartbeat stop, begin resuscitation immediately. (see pp. 18 – 21).

10 Keep casualty covered and place a blanket underneath, if possible.

11 Keep a record of any specimen passed or vomited by the casualty. If possible send samples to the hospital with the casualty.

12 Remove to hospital immediately; transport as a stretcher case, maintaining the treatment position.

Do Not give the casualty anything by mouth.

Forms of revealed internal bleeding and their source

Orifice	How revealed	Description	Possible cause
Nose	Profuse flow	Fresh (bright red) blood	Damage to nasal passages and possible fractured nose.
	Trickle	Straw-coloured fluid (blood mixed with clear cerebro-spinal fluid).	Fractured skull
Ear	Steady bleeding	Fresh (bright-red) blood	Perforated eardrum
	Small trickle of blood	Straw-coloured fluid (blood mixed with clear cerebro-spinal fluid)	Fractured skull
Mouth	Spat out (sputum)	Small amounts of fresh blood	Jaw fracture
	Vomited	Dark-red-brown resembling coffee grounds	Injury to digestive tract, probably bleeding ulcer
	Coughed-up	Fresh (bright-red) blood	Upper airway injury
		Bright-red frothy blood	Injury to lungs caused by rib fracture
Rectum	Steady bleeding	Fresh (bright-red) blood	Piles (haemorrhoids)
	Stool (faeces)	Black tarry consistency	Bleeding from upper intestine
Urethra	Urine	Blood-stained	Bleeding from kidneys or bladder
		Clotted or diluted blood	Injury to urinary tract or bladder (possibly the result of fractured pelvis)
Vagina	Gradual steady bleeding	May be fair to heavy or moderate flow with abdominal cramps.	Severe menstrual bleeding
	Sudden flow	Severe loss, shock and possible history of pregnancy.	Miscarriage or result of abortion

Special Forms of Bleeding

There are a number of wounds and special forms of bleeding where the treatment does not follow the general rules of pressure and/or position of the injured part. Treatment for these wounds is described on the following pages.

Scalp Wounds

Injuries to the scalp most often occur during falls and are particularly common amongst the elderly, ill or intoxicated. Other causes include road traffic accidents, fights, sporting accidents, and falling debris.

Scalp wounds can bleed profusely due to the rich supply of blood to the scalp and because the skin covering the skull is normally tightly stretched. When damaged the skin splits open leaving a gaping wound. This bleeding may appear more alarming than it really is, but there may also be a skull fracture.

Symptoms and Signs
- Pain, tenderness and bleeding of the scalp. Possible lifted flap of scalp.
- Swelling around the wound.
- Possible symptoms and signs of skull fracture (see p. 111).
- Signs of brain damage may be evident (see *Concussion* and *Compression* p. 100).
- Unconsciousness may develop.

Aim
Arrange removal to hospital as *all* head injuries should be examined by a doctor. Control bleeding as soon as possible.

Treatment

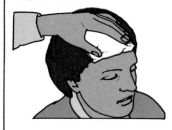

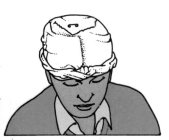

Head bandage

1 Control the bleeding using direct pressure (p. 28). Place a dressing or a pad of material larger than wound, on to it and bandage firmly (see p. 184).

NB The head bandage is *not* intended to apply direct pressure for the control of severe bleeding.

If a fracture or foreign body is present, do not apply heavy direct pressure.

2 If the casualty is conscious lay the casualty down with the head and shoulders slightly raised.

3 Check breathing rate (see p. 12), pulse (see p. 89) and levels of responsiveness (see p. 98) at 10-minute intervals.

4 If the casualty becomes unconscious, place in the Recovery Position with injured side uppermost (see p. 24).

5 If breathing and heartbeat stop, begin resuscitation immediately (see pp. 18 – 21).

6 Remove to hospital immediately. Transport as a stretcher case maintaining the treatment position.

Bleeding from the Ear

Bleeding from inside the ear canal differs from that found in external ear wounds. It generally occurs when an eardrum ruptures or when a skull fracture is present (see p. 72). A perforated eardrum can result from pushing an object into the ear (see p. 159), falling while water-skiing, diving, or being too near an explosion.

Skull fractures are more serious and should be suspected if blood and/or a clear, watery fluid (cerebro-spinal fluid) is issuing from the ear.

Symptoms and signs
If from the eardrum
● Possible pain inside the ear.

● Deafness.
● Moderate flow of blood from the ear.
If from within the skull
● History indicating possible skull fracture (p. 111) or other head injury (see p. 100).
● Casualty complains of a headache.
● Small amounts of blood mixed with clear, watery cerebro-spinal fluid may be coming from the ear.
● Possible unconsciousness.

Aim
Arrange removal to hospital. If skull fracture is suspected pay particular attention to the levels of responsiveness (see p. 98).

Treatment

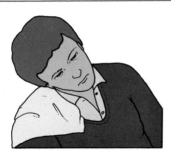

1 Place the conscious casualty in a half-sitting position with the head inclined towards the injured side so that blood or fluid can drain.

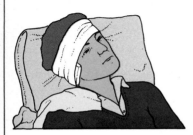

2 Cover the ear with a sterile, unmedicated dressing or similar clean, preferably sterile, material. Secure it very lightly with a bandage or adhesive strapping.

Do Not plug the ear or try to stop the flow from the ear; pressure may build up inside the middle ear.

3 Check breathing rate (see p. 12), pulse (see p. 89) and levels of responsiveness (see p. 98) at 10-minute intervals.

4 To minimise shock, treat as on p. 90.

5 If the casualty becomes unconscious but is breathing normally place in the Recovery Position (see p. 24); the head should lie on the injured side to allow fluid to drain.

6 If breathing and heartbeat stop, begin resuscitation immediately (see pp. 18 – 21).

7 Remove to hospital; transport as a stretcher case maintaining the treatment position.

Nose-bleeds

This is a common condition usually due to bleeding from the blood vessels inside the nostrils. It may occur after a blow to the nose or be the result of sneezing, picking or blowing the nose. However, blood-stained fluid issuing from the nose may be a sign of a fractured skull (see p. 111).

Nose-bleeds can not only involve considerable loss of blood but may also cause the casualty to swallow or inhale a great deal of blood. This may cause vomiting or affect breathing.

Symptoms and Signs
● Moderate flow of blood from nose.
● If skull fracture is present there may be a mixture of blood and clear, watery cerebro-spinal fluid.

Aim
Safeguard the breathing by preventing inhalation of blood and control bleeding.

Treatment

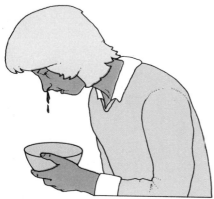

1 Sit the casualty down with the head well forward and loosen any tight clothing around the neck and chest.

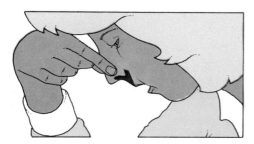

2 Advise the casualty to breathe through the mouth and to pinch the soft part of the nose. (Be prepared to take over if it is tiring for the casualty.)

3 Tell the casualty to spit out any blood in the mouth; swallowed blood may cause nausea and vomiting.

4 Release the pressure after 10 minutes. If the bleeding has not stopped, continue treatment for a further 10 minutes, or as necessary.

Do Not let the casualty raise the head.

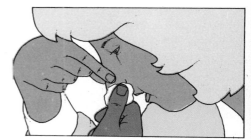

5 While the head is still forward, gently clean around the nose and mouth using a swab or clean dressing soaked in luke-warm water. Do not plug the nose.

6 When the bleeding stops tell the casualty to avoid exertion. Advise the casualty not to blow the nose for at least four hours so as not to disturb the clot.

7 If after 30 minutes the bleeding persists or recurs seek medical aid.

Bleeding Gums

Bleeding from a tooth socket can occur some time after a dental extraction, immediately after accidental loss of a tooth or be associated with jaw fracture (see p. 112). The tearing or knocking out of a tooth generally produces a lacerated mouth wound.

Aim
Safeguard breathing by preventing inhalation of blood and control bleeding. If a tooth has been dislodged seek dental aid.

Symptoms and Signs
● Bleeding from a tooth socket and possible lacerations around the socket.

Treatment

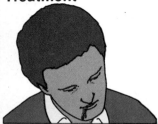

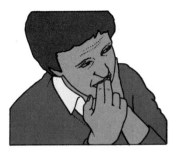

1 Ask the casualty to sit down with the head inclined toward the injured side to allow blood to drain.

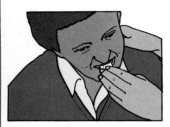

2 Place a thick pad of gauze or a clean cloth on, but *not* into, the bleeding socket.

NB This pad must be thick enough to prevent teeth meeting when the casualty bites on it.

3 Ask the casualty to hold the pad in position with the fingers and then to bite on it for 10 – 20 minutes, supporting the chin on the hand.

4 Tell the casualty to spit out any blood in the mouth while keeping the pad in position; swallowed blood can cause vomiting.

5 After 10 – 20 minutes carefully remove the pad, disturbing the clot as little as possible, and inspect the socket. If it is still bleeding, change the pad and ask the casualty to continue the pressure for a further 10 minutes.

6 Do not wash out the mouth as this may disturb the clot. Advise the casualty to avoid all hot drinks for the next 12 hours.

7 If the bleeding persists or recurs, seek dental or medical aid.

If you suspect jaw fracture treat the casualty as on p. 112.

8 If the casualty has lost a tooth and it can be found, place it in a clean container and seek dental aid as soon as possible. Send the tooth with the casualty.

Mouth Wounds

Cuts in the tongue, lips or lining of the mouth range from trivial injuries to larger wounds. They are usually caused by the casualty's teeth during falls on, or blows to, the face. Bleeding may be severe because the blood supply to this area is rich and the skin covering the blood vessels is very thin.

Symptoms and Signs
- Bleeding in or around the mouth.
- Pain in the affected area.

Aim
Safeguard breathing by preventing the inhalation of blood and control bleeding.

Treatment
1 Ask the casualty to sit down with the head forward and inclined towards the injured side.

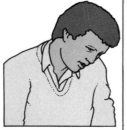

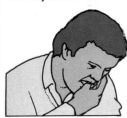

2 To control bleeding, place a clean dressing over the wound and apply direct pressure by squeezing it between thumb and fingers.

3 Tell the casualty to spit out any blood in the mouth; swallowed blood may cause vomiting.

4 If the bleeding persists after 10 – 20 minutes or the wound is large and gaping, remove to hospital.

5 Do not wash out the mouth as this may disturb the clot. Advise the casualty to avoid hot drinks for 12 hours.

Eye Wounds

All eye injuries are potentially serious. Even superficial grazes can lead to scarring of the surface of the eye (cornea) or infection, with possible deterioration of eyesight and even blindness.

The eye can be cut or bruised by direct blows, broken spectacles, or sharp, chipped fragments of metal, grit or glass which fly into it.

For treatment of foreign bodies in the eye, see p. 160.

Symptoms and Signs
- Partial or total loss of vision of the affected eye, even with no visible injury.
- Painful, bloodshot eye, possibly with a visible wound of eyeball or eyelid.
- Loss of blood or clear fluid from the eye wound, possibly with flattening of the normal round contour of the eyeball as the contents leak.

Aim
Protect the eye by preventing movement and seek medical aid.

Treatment
1 Lay the casualty down on the back. Support the head and keep it as still as possible.

Do Not attempt to remove embedded foreign bodies.

2 Ask the casualty to close the injured eye and gently cover it with an eye-pad or a sterile unmedicated dressing. Secure it with a bandage or adhesive plaster.

3 Advise the casualty to keep the sound eye still because movement will cause the injured eye to move. If necessary, bandage both eyes to prevent unnecessary movement. Reassure the casualty before blindfolding.

4 Remove to hospital maintaining the treatment position.

Wounds to the Palm of the Hand

Wounds in the palm can occur when a person handles broken glass or sharp tools or falls on to sharp objects. Such wounds may bleed profusely and can be accompanied by fractures. If the wound is deep, the nerves and tendons in the hand may be damaged.

Symptoms and Signs
- Pain at the site of the wound.
- Profuse bleeding.
- Loss of sensation and movement in the fingers and hand if the underlying nerves and tendons are severed.

Aim
Control bleeding and arrange removal to hospital immediately *without* attempting to remove any embedded foreign bodies.

Treatment

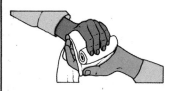
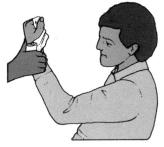

1 To control bleeding, place sterile dressing or gauze and a clean pad over the wound and apply direct pressure (see p. 28). If no dressing or pad is available, use any clean cloth or tissue.

3 Elevate the injured limb.

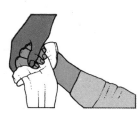
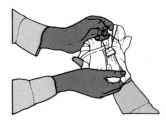

2 Ask casualty to maintain pressure by clenching the fist over the dressing or pad.

If this is not possible, the casualty should grasp the fist of the injured hand with the other hand.

4 Bandage the fist firmly, using the loose ends of the dressing or a folded triangular bandage. Tie off tightly across the knuckles to maintain pressure.

5 Support the arm in an elevation sling (see p. 182).

IF FOREIGN BODY IS PRESENT

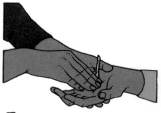

1 Control the bleeding. Apply direct pressure by squeezing the edges of the wound together alongside the foreign body. Treat as on p. 66.

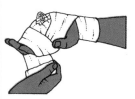

2 Secure dressing with a bandage applied diagonally (see p. 187).

3 Support the arm in an elevation sling (see p. 182).

Abdominal Wounds

A deep wound of the abdominal wall is serious not only because it will involve external bleeding but also because the underlying organs may have been punctured or lacerated. Either can result in severe internal bleeding and possible infection. Part of the intestine may also be protruding from the wound.

Symptoms and Signs
● General abdominal pain.
● Bleeding and associated wounds in the abdominal area.
● Part of the intestine may be visible in, or protruding from, the wound.
● Casualty may be vomiting.
● Symptoms and signs of shock (see p. 90).

Aim
Minimise infection and control bleeding while preventing protrusion of the intestines. Arrange urgent removal to hospital.

Treatment

1 Control any bleeding by carefully squeezing the edges of the wound together.

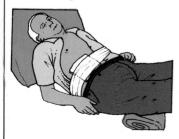

2 Place the casualty in a half-sitting position with the knees bent up to prevent the wound gaping and reduce strain on the injured area. Support the shoulders and the knees.

3 Apply a dressing to the wound and secure with a bandage or adhesive strapping.

4 If the casualty becomes unconscious but is breathing normally, support the abdomen and place the casualty in the Recovery Position (see p. 24).

5 If breathing and heartbeat stop, begin resuscitation immediately (see pp. 18 – 21).

6 To minimise shock, treat as on p. 90.

Do Not give the casualty anything by mouth.

7 Check breathing rate (see p. 12) and pulse (see p. 89) at 10-minute intervals. Look for evidence of internal bleeding (see p. 72).

8 If the casualty coughs or vomits support the abdomen by pressing gently on the cloth or dressing to prevent protrusion of the intestines.

9 Remove to hospital immediately. Transport as a stretcher case maintaining the treatment position.

IF PART OF THE INTESTINE PROTRUDES FROM THE WOUND

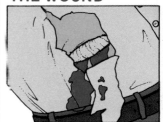

1 Control bleeding (see p. 28) but avoid heavy direct pressure.

Do Not touch the protruding intestines.

2 Cover with a *damp* sterile dressing or clean cloth secured with a loose bandage.

If the casualty coughs or vomits, support the wound as in step 8.

3 Position and treat casualty as left.

Penetrating Chest and Back Wounds

Chest and back injuries caused by a sharp knife or gunshot penetrating the body or ribs being forced outwards through the skin allow air directly into the chest cavity. These wounds can become complicated and may develop into "sucking wounds".

In these injuries, the lung on the affected side deflates, even if it is not punctured, and is unable to take in air. In addition, as the ribs rise when the casualty breathes in, air is sucked in through the wound filling the chest cavity and impairing the action of the sound lung. The amount of oxygen reaching the bloodstream may be insufficient and asphyxia may result (see p. 45).

Symptoms and Signs
● Casualty has pain in the chest.
● Difficulty in breathing; breaths are shallow due to air in the chest cavity.
● Blueness of the mouth, nailbeds and skin (cyanosis) indicating onset of significant asphyxia.
● Coughed-up, bright-red, frothy blood if lung is injured.
● The sound of air being sucked into the chest may be heard when the casualty is breathing in.
● Blood-stained liquid bubbling from the chest wound during breathing out.
● Symptoms and signs of shock (see p. 90).

Aim
Ease breathing by immediately sealing the wound. Arrange urgent removal to hospital.

Treatment

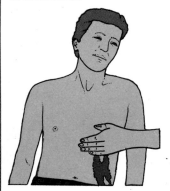

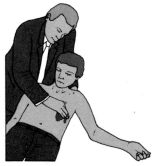

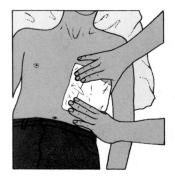

1 Immediately seal the open wound with the palm of your hand.

2 Place the casualty in a half-sitting position with the head and shoulders supported; incline the body towards the injured side so that the sound lung is uppermost.

3 Gently cover the wound with a sterile unmedicated dressing as soon as possible.

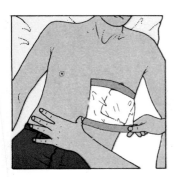

4 If possible, form an airtight seal by covering the dressing with a plastic sheet or metal foil. Secure and seal the edges of the dressing with layers of adhesive tape, strapping and/or a bandage.

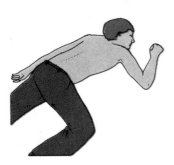

5 If the casualty becomes unconscious but is breathing normally, place in the Recovery Position with the sound lung uppermost (see p. 24).

6 To minimise shock, treat as on p. 90.

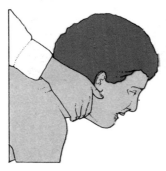

7 Check breathing rate (see p. 12), pulse (see p. 89) and levels of responsiveness (see p. 98) at 10-minute intervals. Look for evidence of internal bleeding (see p. 72).

8 Remove to hospital immediately; transport as a stretcher case maintaining the treatment position.

IF A FOREIGN BODY IS PRESENT

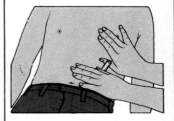

1 Seal the wound, by squeezing the edges of the wound alongside the foreign body.

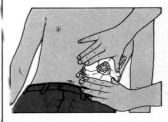

2 Pack gauze or a clean cloth around the foreign body and use a ring pad, if immediately available (see p. 66).

3 Position and treat the casualty as steps 4 to 8, left.

Vaginal Bleeding

This can be severe menstrual bleeding or the result of a miscarriage or internal injury; the history of the condition is essential to the diagnosis of the emergency. If you suspect a miscarriage treat as described on p. 210. Heavy menstrual bleeding or miscarriage may also be accompanied by severe cramps. These normally occur at the beginning of the period but may last for several days.

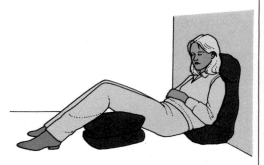

Symptoms and Signs
● Moderate to severe bleeding from the vagina.
● Symptoms and signs of shock may be present (see p. 90).
● Cramp-like pains in the lower abdomen or pelvic area.

Aim
Reassure casualty and if in doubt about the severity of the bleeding, arrange removal to hospital.

Treatment
1 If possible, remove the woman to a place which has some privacy or arrange for screening. Give her a sanitary dressing, if available, or a clean towel to place over the entrance of the vagina.

2 Lay the woman down with the head and shoulders slightly raised and the knees bent, supported on a blanket. (This will relax the abdominal muscles.)

3 If the pains are severe, and obviously due to menstruation, the casualty may be allowed to take one or two of her own pain-killing tablets or those made specifically for the relief of menstrual cramps.

4 If bleeding continues and is severe, minimise shock by treating as on p. 90. Arrange removal to hospital immediately; maintain the treatment position.

Bleeding Varicose Veins

Certain veins in the legs contain numerous cup-like non-return valves to keep the blood flowing back to the heart. When these valves deteriorate, the blood tends to pool and the veins become swollen and protruding or "varicosed". Because the leg veins are large and contain a large volume of blood when varicosed, a sudden massive blood loss can occur when they are injured or burst. If such bleeding is not controlled immediately the condition can be fatal.

Symptoms and Signs
● Severe external bleeding; blood will be dark-red.
● Symptoms and signs of shock (see p. 90).
● Unconsciousness may develop.

Aim
Control bleeding by using direct pressure and arrange removal to hospital immediately.

Treatment

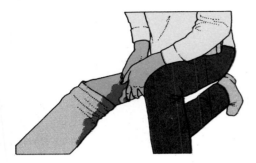

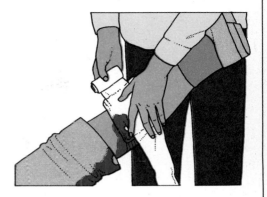

1 Immediately expose wound and apply direct pressure by pressing with fingers or palm of hand (see p. 28).

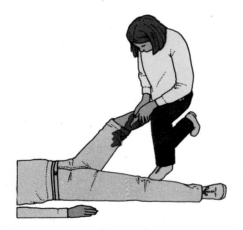

2 Lay the casualty on the back and raise the injured leg as high as possible to encourage the blood to return to the heart.

3 Remove any constricting clothing such as elastic-topped or support stockings, garters or tights which may be impeding blood flow back to heart.

4 Place a sterile, unmedicated dressing over the wound. It should be large enough to cover the whole area around the bleeding varicose vein. Tie bandage firmly enough to control bleeding but not so tight as to cut off circulation (see p. 128).

If no suitable dressing is available, place a piece of gauze over the wound, cover it with a pad of cotton wool and bandage firmly. Alternatively make an improvised dressing (see p. 175).

If bleeding does not stop and bandages are soaked with blood, apply further dressings or pads and bandages on top of the original ones.

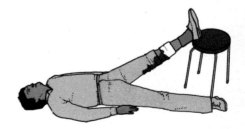

5 Keep the leg raised and supported.

6 To minimise shock, treat as on p. 90.

7 Remove to hospital maintaining the treatment position.

Crush Injuries

These injuries often involve damage to a great deal of skin, muscle and bone and medical aid should always be sought. There may be serious external and internal bleeding. In particular, there may be damage to the blood vessels supplying a limb, therefore, if release and rescue are delayed, the part may be lost due to a prolonged lack of oxygenated blood. In some cases where the part remains crushed for more than an hour, serum will pour into the injured tissues causing them to become swollen and hard, blood pressure will fall and shock may develop. There will also be an accumulation of toxic chemicals within the body because of substances released by damaged muscle. On release from crushing, these substances can flood back to the rest of the body causing kidney failure which can be fatal.

Therefore, although a casualty may show little sign of injury when released, except redness and swelling, a serious condition may be present.

Symptoms and Signs

● Crushed limb may be tingling or numb.
● Swollen and hard tissue around injured part because serum from the blood has poured into the area.
● Bruising and formation of blisters at the site of injury.
● General symptoms and signs of fracture (see p. 108).
● Crushed or trapped limb will be cool, pale and pulseless if arteries are compressed.
● Symptoms and signs of shock (see p. 90).

Aim

Prevent damage to the kidneys caused by the release of toxic chemicals. In all cases where a casualty has been trapped with a crushed limb for longer than 30 minutes call the emergency services *before* attempting release.

Treatment

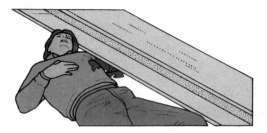

1 Control serious bleeding and treat any wounds; immobilise fractures as far as possible (see pp. 106–127).

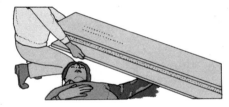

2 If the trapped limb can be released without delay, remove the weight. Keep casualty lying down with the head low and legs raised where possible. Advise casualty not to move.

NB Record time of release and duration of crushing.

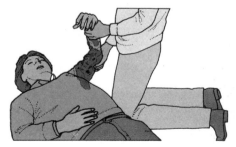

3 Immobilise the affected limb using pillows and rolled-up clothing or blankets, and if injuries allow, elevate limb. Where possible, crush injuries should be left uncovered.

4 To minimise shock, treat as on p. 90.

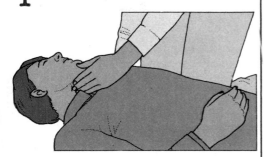

5 Check breathing rate (see p. 12), pulse (see p. 89) and levels of responsiveness (see p. 98) at 10-minute intervals.

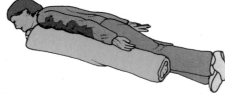

6 If the casualty becomes unconscious but is breathing normally, place in the Recovery Position (see p. 24).

7 If breathing and heartbeat stop, begin resuscitation immediately (see pp. 18–21).

8 Remove to hospital immediately. Transport as a stretcher case maintaining the treatment position; notify ambulance crew of duration of crushing.

If removal to hospital will be delayed by more than 30 minutes and internal injury is *not* suspected, give the casualty sips of cold water.

NB If the crush injury is short-lived and only involves the fingers, hand or foot, place the injured part under cold running water or apply a cold compress (see p. 176).

Bruises

A bruise consists of internal bleeding from damaged blood vessels which seeps through the tissues, and appears as a discoloration under the skin. A heavy fall on fleshy parts of the body such as the hip and buttocks, can result in considerable internal bleeding.

Symptoms and Signs
- Pain and swelling in the affected area.
- Bluish-purple discoloration at site of injury.
- Pattern bruising, in which outlines of clothing worn is seen in bruise. This should be regarded as a potentially dangerous sign as it may indicate damage to internal organs.

Aim
Slow down blood flow by cooling.

Treatment
1 Raise and support the injured part in the position the casualty finds most comfortable.

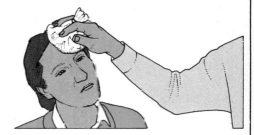

2 Apply a cold compress to the injured area (see p. 176) to restrict bleeding and reduce swelling.

3 If in doubt about the severity of the injury, seek medical aid.

Animal Bites

Germs are harboured in the mouths of both domestic and wild animals. Animals have sharp, pointed teeth. Because of this their bites often leave deep puncture wounds and germs may be injected deep into the tissues. Human bites are also potentially dangerous.

Any bite causing a break in the skin needs prompt attention to prevent infection. It may be complicated by tetanus (see p. 69) and in some countries rabies (see below). Savaging by a dog may also result in multiple lacerations.

Symptoms and Signs
● One or more small puncture wounds in the pattern of the teeth.
● A number of lacerations indicating a tearing bite.
● Bleeding can be severe or may be slight, depending on the extent of injury.

Aim
Treat the wound and seek medical aid: arrange urgent removal to hospital if wound is serious. Dog bites should be reported to the police.

Treatment
FOR SUPERFICIAL BITES

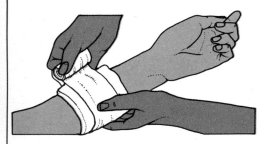

1 Wash wound thoroughly with soapy water for 5 minutes. Dry it and cover with a sterile unmedicated dressing.

2 Seek medical aid.

FOR SERIOUS WOUNDS

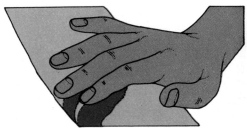

1 Control any serious bleeding with direct pressure and dress wound (see p. 28).

2 Cover with a sterile unmedicated dressing and bandage securely.

3 Remove to hospital.

RABIES
Rabies is a potentially fatal condition spread by the saliva of infected animals. Although not currently found in the United Kingdom, rabies is endemic in many countries. Therefore, if an animal bite is sustained in a foreign country or if you suspect an infected animal may have been smuggled into the British Isles, you *must* make sure that the casualty has a course of injections.

To confirm or exclude a rabies infection, the animal must be examined medically. If possible, attempt to isolate the animal, *without* endangering yourself. If the animal escapes, notify the police immediately.

Snake Bites

The only poisonous snake native to the British Isles is the adder. However, there are many poisonous snakes kept as pets, some of which may escape or attack their owners. In addition to the injuries produced by a bite, fright resulting in severe shock may also be evident.

In countries where there are numerous dangerous snakes, it is important to identify the snake so that appropriate anti-venom serum can be administered. Therefore, either record its description or, if it has been captured or killed, keep it. Colour and markings are the best guide, but in general, poisonous snakes have slit eyes and the non-poisonous snakes have rounded ones.

Symptoms and Signs
- Casualty may experience disturbed vision.
- Casualty may feel nauseated or already be vomiting.

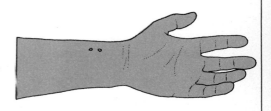

- One or two small puncture wounds with sharp pain and local swelling.
- Breathing may become difficult or fail altogether.
- Symptoms and signs of shock (see p. 90).
- Salivation and sweating may appear in advanced stages of venom reaction.

Aim
Reassure the casualty, prevent movement to delay the absorption of venom, and arrange immediate removal to hospital. Identify the snake and, if possible, take it to the hospital in a safe container, along with the casualty.

Treatment

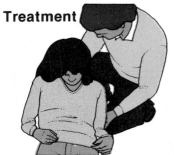

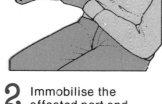

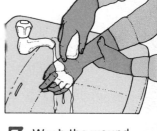

1 Lay the casualty down and advise not to move.

2 Immobilise the affected part and keep it below the level of the heart.

3 Wash the wound thoroughly with soap and water, if available.

4 If the casualty becomes unconscious but is breathing normally, place in the Recovery Position (see p. 24).

5 If breathing and heartbeat stop, begin resuscitation immediately (see p. 18 – 21).

6 Remove the casualty to hospital. Take the snake, if possible, in a safe container.

CIRCULATORY DISORDERS

Blood is circulated around the body by the heart through blood vessels to the tissues and cells of the body, before returning via the heart to the lungs where it is reoxygenated. (See *Blood and the Circulation* pp. 26 – 7)

There are several factors which can affect circulation: the volume and quality of the blood in the system, the pressure at which it is circulated, and the condition of the heart and the vessels through which the blood flows.

The average adult has 6 litres (10 pints) of blood circulating in the body. The composition of the blood is vital to the health of the tissues. Normal blood consists of a transparent yellow fluid called plasma in which red cells, white cells and blood platelets are suspended. The coloured pigment in the red cells (haemoglobin) carries oxygen to the tissues. The white cells engulf and remove any harmful bodies in the tissues, such as germs and dead cells, and the platelets assist the blood to clot.

The pressure at which blood flows is determined by the force required to make sure all the blood reaches the tissues. If it is too low, due to severe loss of blood volume for example, then the vital organs receive a reduced supply of blood and cannot function properly and shock may develop.

Blood will continue to flow around the body and will only clot if it escapes from damaged blood vessels (see *Wounds and Bleeding* p. 64). However, in one form of circulatory condition, thrombosis, clotting may occur within a blood vessel – this can block the vessel concerned and so cut off vital supplies of oxygenated blood. Clots may lodge where they form, or be carried around the body until they block an important artery.

Hardened arteries are another cause of circulatory disorder. Continually raised blood pressure (which is more common as age increases) can cause arteries to rupture resulting in internal bleeding. The most common example of this is a cerebral haemorrhage (a form of stroke) and it occurs when a cerebral artery which supplies the brain, ruptures and blood leaks into brain tissue.

Poor blood circulation, possibly aggravated by the slowing-down process of old age, can contribute to thrombosis

Head and upper body

Lungs

Heart

Liver

Legs and lower body

Kidneys

Intestines

as can the presence of narrowed blood vessels which may also have "fatty" deposits on their walls. Clots carried up into the arteries of the brain can cause a stroke (cerebral thrombosis); clots in the lungs may interrupt the normal blood flow and therefore the oxygenation process (pulmonary embolism); clots which form in the coronary arteries of the heart itself cause heart attacks (coronary thrombosis).

The heart muscle contracts and relaxes in the same way as other muscles and has its own separate blood supply, the coronary arteries. Unlike other muscles, however, it must function continuously in order to sustain all the other organs of the body – even if its own oxygen supply is reduced

The coronary arteries can, like all other arteries, become narrowed with age so that the amount of blood able to pass through them to the heart is reduced. The more heart muscle that is affected by this lack of blood, the less efficient the heart becomes; the beat will become weak and/or irregular and eventually it may stop altogether (cardiac arrest).

The Pulse

This is the wave of pressure which passes along the arteries indicating the pumping action of the heart. It can be felt at any place where an artery is close to the surface of the body and can be pressed against a bone.

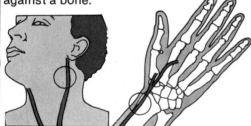

Carotid pulse   Radial pulse

The most useful pulse, the carotid pulse, can be felt just below the angle of the jaw in the hollow between the voice box and the adjoining muscle (see p. 17). However, unless cardiac arrest is suspected, the pulse is usually taken at the wrist on the thumb and palm side just above the crease where the artery runs along the inner side of the forearm bone (radial pulse). Slip your fingers into the hollow just above the bottom end of the bone and press your finger-tips lightly over the artery (do not use your thumb because it has a pulse of its own). To take the pulse, use a watch with a second hand and count the number of beats in a minute.

The three things to check and record are: the rate, strength and rhythm. Note whether it is fast or slow, strong or feeble, or regular or irregular. The average pulse rate in an adult is 72 beats per minute but it can vary between 60 and 80. It increases during stress, exercise, some illnesses, while taking alcohol, or as a result of injury. The pulse rate in elderly persons and some athletes may be slower (between 50 and 60 beats per minute), and it is faster in young babies (about 120 beats per minute).

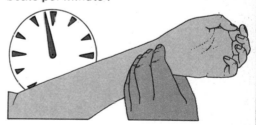

A normal pulse is regular and strong. An abnormality such as a weak or pounding pulse may indicate an abnormal state in a casualty. For example, a fast, weak pulse in an apparently uninjured person could indicate that there is concealed internal loss of blood or fluid and that the heart is having to work much faster to circulate a lower volume of blood.

Shock

This is a condition of general bodily weakness resulting from some form of injury or illness which has reduced the volume of blood or fluid in the body. It can vary from faintness to complete collapse. Commonly referred to as "Traumatic" (injury) shock, this is a serious condition which may prove fatal even when the casualty's injuries have been adequately treated.

Shock can be caused by the following examples of blood/fluid loss: loss of blood by external or internal bleeding; loss of plasma from major burns; loss of water due to intestinal obstruction; recurrent vomiting or severe diarrhoea; acute abdominal emergencies; or a heart attack. Extreme pain or fear can produce a similar state.

Symptoms and Signs

The body reacts to shock by directing more blood to the arteries supplying the vital organs (e.g., brain, heart and kidneys) at the expense of those supplying the less important tissues (e.g., muscle and skin). As the casualty's condition deteriorates the symptoms and signs will become more pronounced.

● Casualty will feel weak, faint and giddy and be anxious and restless.
● Casualty may feel sick and may vomit.
● Casualty could feel thirsty.
● Skin becomes pale, cold and clammy and sweating might develop.
● Breathing can be shallow and rapid; casualty may be yawning and sighing.
● Pulse rate increases but becomes weaker and sometimes irregular as blood/fluid volume drops.
● Unconsciousness may develop.
● There may be evidence of associated external or internal injury.

Aim

Ensure an adequate blood supply to the heart, lungs and brain. Determine the cause of the shock, treat it and arrange removal to hospital.

Treatment

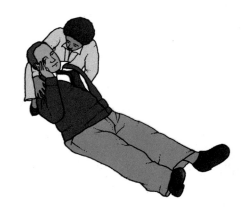

1 Immediately reassure and comfort the casualty.

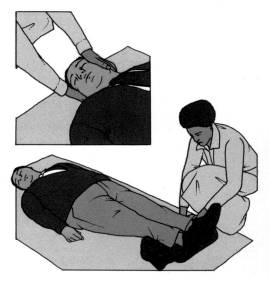

2 If the casualty's condition allows, lay the casualty down on the back on a blanket. Keep the head low and turned on one side (to maintain blood supply to the brain and to lessen the dangers of vomiting e.g., stomach contents entering windpipe and causing asphyxia). Raise legs unless you suspect leg fractures.

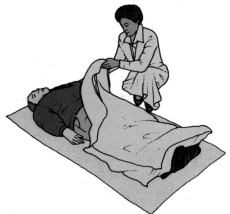

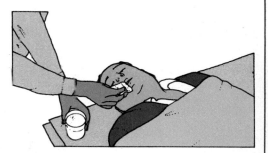

6 If the casualty complains of thirst, moisten lips with water but do not give anything to drink.

3 Keep the casualty warm. Cover the casualty with a blanket.

Do Not apply a hot water bottle — this will increase the

blood flow to the vessels of the skin and take it away from the vital organs.

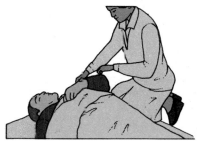

7 Check breathing rate (see p. 12), pulse (see p. 89) and levels of responsiveness (see p. 98) at 10-minute intervals.

8 If the casualty's breathing becomes difficult, if vomiting seems likely or if the casualty becomes unconscious, place in the Recovery Position (see p. 24).

9 If breathing and heartbeat stop, begin resuscitation immediately (see pp. 18 – 21).

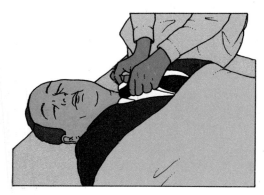

4 Loosen any tight clothing to help the circulation and assist breathing.

5 Search for and, if possible, treat the cause of the shock.

10 Remove to hospital immediately. Transport as a stretcher case maintaining the treatment position.

NB

Do Not move the casualty unnecessarily — this

will increase shock.

Do Not give the casualty anything by mouth — it

will prevent or delay the subsequent administration of an anaesthetic.

Do Not let the casualty smoke.

Fainting

A faint is a brief loss of consciousness — generally of no more than a few minutes duration — caused by a temporary reduction in the flow of blood to the brain. Recovery is usually rapid and complete.

It may be a nervous reaction to pain or fright; or the result of an emotional upset, exhaustion, or lack of food. It is, however, more common after long periods of physical inactivity where lack of muscular activity causes a large volume of blood to collect in the lower part of the body and legs, thus reducing the amount of blood available for the rest of the circulation.

Symptoms and Signs
These are the same as for early stages of shock (see p. 90), but:
● Pulse will be SLOW and weak (this is the important clue).
● The casualty may look very pale.

Aim
Position the casualty so that gravity helps increase the flow of blood to the brain.

Treatment

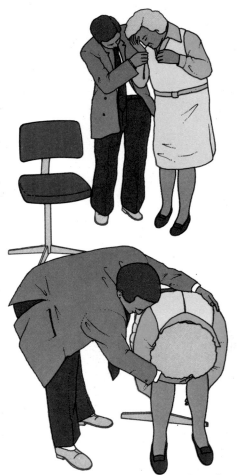

1 If the casualty feels unsteady, sit the casualty down and help to lean forward with the head between the knees, and advise to take deep breaths.

If on parade or standing in a crowd, advise the casualty to flex the leg muscles and toes to aid circulation.

If the casualty is unconscious, but breathing normally, lay down with legs raised or place in the Recovery Position (see p. 24). Maintain an open airway (see p. 15).

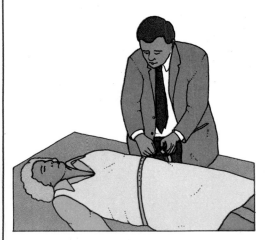

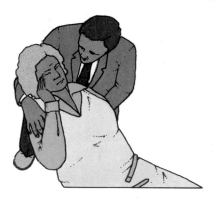

2 Loosen any tight clothing at the neck, chest and waist, to assist circulation and breathing.

3 Make sure that the casualty has plenty of fresh air: place casualty in a current of fresh air and fan air on to the face. If necessary, place casualty in the shade.

4 Check for and treat any injury that the casualty has sustained on falling.

6 Reassure casualty whilst regaining conscicusness; gradually raise to a sitting position.

If in doubt about the casualty's condition, seek medical aid.

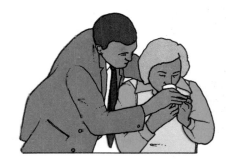

Do Not give the casualty anything by mouth until fully conscious and then only sips of cold water.

Do Not give the casualty any alcohol.

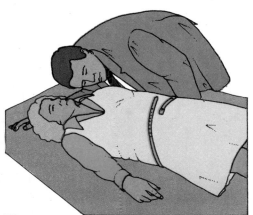

5 Check breathing rate (see p. 12), pulse (see p. 89) and levels of responsiveness (see p. 98) at 10-minute intervals.

Heart Attacks

Sudden interference with the normal action of the heart will have serious consequences. This can occur if a blood clot blocks a coronary artery preventing blood reaching the heart muscle (coronary obstruction/thrombosis), or because the heart is stopped for another reason (cardiac arrest).

CORONARY OBSTRUCTION
Symptoms and Signs
● Sudden, crushing, vice-like pain in the centre of the chest (sometimes described as severe indigestion) which may spread to the arms, throat, jaw or back.

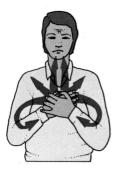

● Sudden dizziness or giddiness causing the casualty to sit down or lean against a wall for support.
● Skin may be ashen; lips and extremities may become blue (cyanosis).
● Profuse sweating may develop.
● Breathlessness can occur.
● Fast pulse which becomes weaker and may become irregular.
● Symptoms and signs of shock (see p. 90).
● Unconsciousness may develop.
● Breathing and heartbeat may stop.

Aim
Minimise the work of the heart by placing the casualty in an appropriate resting position. Arrange removal to hospital immediately, making it clear to the ambulance service that a heart attack is suspected. Be prepared to resuscitate.

Treatment

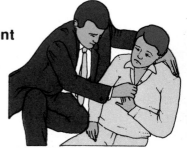

1 If conscious, gently support and place the casualty in a half-sitting position with head and shoulders supported and knees bent.

Do Not allow the casualty to move unnecessarily as this will put extra strain on the heart.

2 Loosen any constricting clothing around neck, chest and waist.

3 If the casualty becomes unconscious but is breathing normally, place in the Recovery Position (see p. 24).

4 If breathing and heartbeat stop, begin resuscitation immediately (see pp. 18 – 21).

5 To minimise shock, treat as on p. 90.

6 Check breathing rate (see p. 12), pulse (see p. 89) and levels of responsiveness (see p. 98) at 10-minute intervals.

7 Remove to hospital immediately. Transport as a stretcher case maintaining the treatment position.

CARDIAC ARREST

This is a very serious condition in which the heart suddenly stops beating altogether. It can be the result of an extensive coronary obstruction.

Symptoms and Signs
- The casualty becomes unconscious.
- No pulse can be felt at neck.

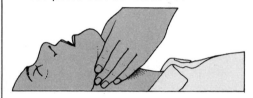

- Breathing and heartbeat will cease.
- Skin becomes ashen.

Aim
Attempt to revive the casualty by commencing resuscitation without delay. Arrange removal to hospital, making it clear that a heart attack is suspected.

Treatment
1 Begin resuscitation immediately. (see p. 18 – 21).

2 Remove to hospital immediately. If necessary, continue resuscitation on the way to hospital.

Angina Pectoris

Severe pains in the chest, often mistaken for a coronary obstruction, occur when the coronary arteries, which supply blood to the heart, become too narrow for sufficient oxygenated blood to reach the muscles of the heart.

This condition is common in the elderly and is usually brought on by overexertion during exercise, and sometimes by excitement. Normally these attacks only last a few minutes and the pain will stop if the casualty rests.

Symptoms and Signs
- Pain in chest often spreading down the left shoulder to arm and fingers. (It may also spread to the casualty's throat and jaw and across to the other arm.)

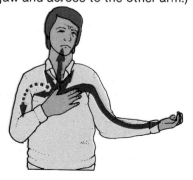

- Skin may be ashen and lips may be blue.
- Casualty may be short of breath.
- General weakness.

Aim
Place the casualty in a resting position in which the heart is able to work most effectively.

Treatment
1 Help the casualty to sit down. Support in this position by placing a blanket or jacket behind casualty, and padding under the knees.

2 Reassure the casualty and advise to rest. Loosen clothing around neck, chest and waist.

NB Many people who suffer from Angina Pectoris carry special medicine with them for the prevention or treatment of an attack. Glyceryl trinitrate is commonly prescribed and often absorbed by placing under the tongue.

3 If symptoms persist, arrange removal to hospital.

Stroke

This term is used to describe a condition in which the blood supply to part of the brain is suddenly and critically impaired by a blood clot (cerebral thrombosis) or when a ruptured artery leaks blood into the brain (cerebral haemorrhage). The latter is more likely in people who have high blood pressure. In either case, the affected brain cells cease to function altogether.

Each area of the brain controls a different system or part of the body, and any deficiency resulting from a stroke depends on how much, and which part, of the brain is affected. Major strokes are often fatal, but many people make successful recoveries from minor strokes. Strokes are more common in people over 55, in those who are known to suffer from blackouts or circulatory disorders or in those who have had previous strokes. The symptoms and signs may be confused with drunkenness.

Symptoms and Signs
- Sudden severe headache.
- A full, bounding pulse.
- Casualty is disorientated and confused, and may be anxious and weeping.
- Giddiness and possible unconsciousness.

Depending on the extent of the stroke, one or more of the following physical defects may be also apparent:
- Paralysis of mouth — the corner of the mouth may droop, saliva may dribble from it, and speech may be slurred.
- Weakness and decreased sensation in one or both limbs and on one side of the body.
- Flushed face with hot, dry skin.

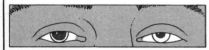

- Pupils may be unequally dilated.
- Loss of bladder and bowel control.

Aim
In general, First Aid for a stroke is supportive. Be prepared for unconsciousness to develop and/or deepen at any time. Keep the airway open and begin resuscitation, if necessary. Arrange removal to hospital as soon as possible.

Treatment
1 If conscious, lay the casualty down with head and shoulders slightly raised and supported. Position head on the side to allow saliva to drain from the mouth.

2 Loosen any constricting clothing around the neck, chest and waist to assist circulation and breathing.

3 To minimise shock, treat as on p. 90.

Do Not give casualty anything by mouth.

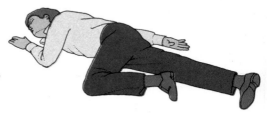

4 If casualty becomes unconscious place in the Recovery Position (see p. 24).

5 If breathing and heartbeat stop, begin resuscitation immediately, (see pp. 18 – 21).

6 Remove the casualty to hospital immediately. Transport as a stretcher case maintaining the treatment position.

UNCONSCIOUSNESS

The movements and functions of the body and the levels of responsiveness are governed by the nervous system.

Partial consciousness or unconsciousness in a casualty indicates that there is an interruption of the normal activity of the brain which can be dangerous to the casualty. There are many causes of unconsciousness, the most common of which are: head injury, fainting, heart attack, stroke, asphyxia, epilepsy, shock, poisoning, infantile convulsions and diabetes. Treatment for most of these conditions can be found in this chapter.

THE NERVOUS SYSTEM

This system comprises the brain, spinal cord and nerves.

The brain is an extremely delicate structure made up of a mass of nerve cells. It is here that sensations are analysed and orders are given to the muscles. The brain is encased in the skull and suspended in clear (cerebro-spinal) fluid, which acts as a partial shock absorber. Nonetheless, since it is free to move within the skull, the brain is sensitive to violent movement or pressure.

The spinal cord is a mass of nerve fibres extending from the brain through an opening in the base of the skull. The cord runs down through the neck and the spinal column (see p. 114).

The peripheral nerves emerge in pairs, each containing motor and sensory nerves, from the brain and spinal cord. Sensory nerves transport impressions received by the senses (sight, hearing, touch, etc.) to the brain and motor nerves then transport the "orders" given by the brain to the voluntary muscles (those under the control of the will, see p. 128). When a nerve is cut, there is a loss of feeling, power and movement in that part of the body controlled by the damaged nerve.

If the body is subjected to a harmful stimulus, such as when touching a hot object, a "reflex action" will attempt to remove the affected part of the body from the stimulus quickly by by-passing the normal pathway to and from the brain.

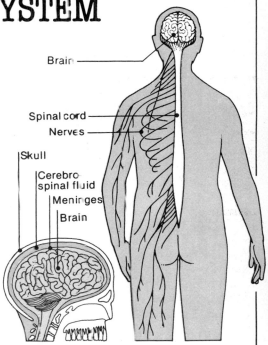

Brain

Spinal cord
Nerves

Skull
Cerebro-spinal fluid
Meninges
Brain

THE AUTONOMIC SYSTEM

This is the network of nerves which controls the involuntary muscles — the muscles which regulate the vital functions of the body such as circulation, respiration and digestion. This system is not controlled by the will, and acts continuously whether a person is awake or asleep.

The Unconscious Casualty

Unconsciousness is the result of an interference with the functions of the brain. The seriousness of the condition can be gauged by testing the casualty's response to stimuli such as sound or touch.

It is important to take note of any change in the casualty's condition because it will govern the treatment eventually given. A casualty may progress through any of the stages outlined below – either improving or deteriorating.

If possible, a written report of the levels of responsiveness should be given to the doctor or ambulance crew. If you are on your own, this report will have to wait until you have treated the casualty or casualties and are waiting for skilled help to arrive. If there are any bystanders, they can be used to keep a record while you treat the casualty or casualties.

NB For examining the unconscious casualty see *Examination* pp. 36 – 40.

Aim

To find out the cause of the condition and treat it as quickly as possible. Seek medical aid or arrange removal to hospital.

LEVELS OF RESPONSIVENESS

These are the stages through which a casualty may pass during progression from consciousness to unconsciousness or vice versa.
The casualty may:

1 Respond normally to questions and conversation.

2 Only answer direct questions.

3 Respond only vaguely to questions.

4 Obey commands.

5 Only respond to pain.

6 Not respond at all.

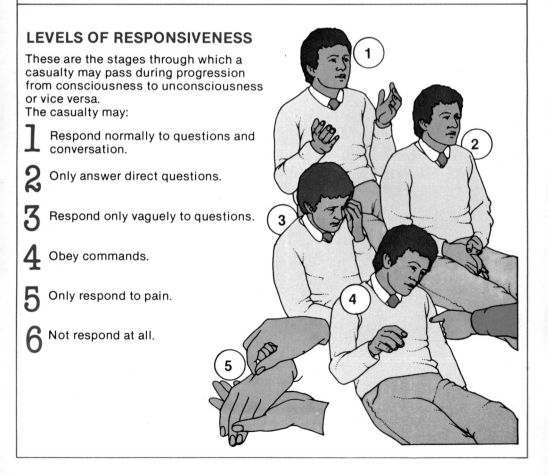

General Treatment

1 Ensure that the casualty's air passages are open. Remove any loose dentures or detached teeth and clear the casualty's mouth of any vomit or blood. Loosen any constricting clothing around the neck, chest and waist.

2 If breathing becomes difficult or stops, begin Artificial Ventilation immediately (see p. 18).

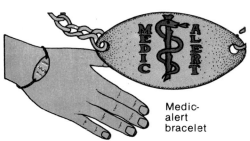

Medic-
alert
bracelet

3 Conduct a thorough examination of the casualty to determine the cause of unconsciousness (see Examination pp. 36 – 40); look carefully for signs of head injury and any warning bracelets, lockets or cards (see p. 41).

4 Treat any serious wounds and fractures.

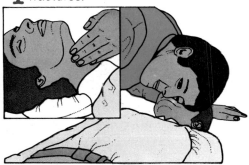

5 Establish level of responsiveness, check pulse (see p. 89) and breathing rate (see p. 12) and record any observations.

6 If the casualty is breathing normally, place in the Recovery Position (see p. 24).

NB If there is any possibility of spinal injury do not move the casualty unless difficulty in breathing makes it vital.

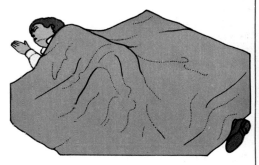

7 Cover the casualty with a blanket and, if possible, place another blanket underneath.

8 If removal to hospital will be delayed, continue to check the levels of responsiveness, pulse (see p. 89) and breathing rate (see p. 12) at 10-minute intervals and keep a written record for the doctor.

Do Not give an unconscious casualty anything by mouth.

Do Not leave the casualty unattended.

If a casualty recovers consciousness, reassure and observe; advise the casualty to see a doctor.

Head Injuries

Head injuries can result in damage to, or disturbance of, the brain. If this occurs, then consciousness may be clouded or lost, concussion or compression may result and other associated injuries or conditions may be masked. A thorough examination of the casualty is, therefore, essential (see pp. 36–40).

Direct blows to the head, heavy enough to cause scalp wounds or bruising, may be accompanied by skull fractures. This type of injury must, therefore, receive urgent medical attention (see *Skull fracture* p. 111, and *Scalp wound* p. 73). With thin skulls, a fracture may be present with little evidence of external damage.

These injuries are common results of: falls, particularly in the elderly, ill or intoxicated; road accidents; sporting activities; or day-to-day work in high-risk occupations such as construction work or mining.

CONCUSSION

This is a condition of widespread but temporary disturbance of the brain sometimes described as "brain-shaking". It can result from a blow to the head, a fall from a height on to the feet or a blow on the point of the jaw.

This condition can occur *without* apparent unconsciousness. In some cases unconsciousness may have been so brief that the casualty may be unaware of, or have forgotten, the initial incident. However, because concussion can precede compression (see opposite), it is important to observe the casualty closely after any incident involving injury to the head. If symptoms persist or the casualty's condition deteriorates, refer to a doctor without delay.

Symptoms and Signs
● Brief or partial loss of consciousness.
While the casualty is unconscious
● Breathing may be shallow.
● Face may be pale.
● Skin may be cold and clammy.
● Pulse may be rapid and weak.
During recovery
● Casualty may feel nauseated or already be vomiting.
On recovering consciousness
● Casualty may not remember any events just before or after the incident.

NB If unconsciousness persists, suspect compression.

Aim
Treat unconsciousness and any obvious wounds and seek medical aid.

Treatment
1 In mild cases, place the casualty in the care of a responsible person and advise the casualty to consult a doctor.

2 Carry out the general treatment for the unconscious casualty where it is relevant.

3 To minimise shock treat as on p. 90.

4 In serious cases check breathing rate (see p. 12), pulse (see p. 89) and levels of responsiveness; watch carefully for signs of compression (see opposite) even after the casualty has apparently recovered.

5 If the casualty was unconscious for a short time or you are in doubt about the casualty's condition, arrange removal to hospital.

COMPRESSION

This is a very serious condition in which pressure is exerted on the brain by blood accumulating within the skull or by pressure from bone in a depressed fracture (see p. 111). Compression can follow concussion and it may develop up to 48 hours after the casualty has apparently recovered.

Symptoms and Signs
- Breathing becomes noisy.
- Body temperature may rise; face becomes flushed but remains dry.
- Pulse is full and bounding but slow.
- Pupils may be different sizes.

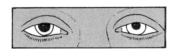

- There may be weakness or paralysis of one side of the body.

NB As compression develops the casualty's level of responsiveness falls

Aim
Arrange removal to hospital immediately. This condition requires urgent medical treatment.

Treatment
1 Carry out the general treatment for the unconscious casualty.

2 Remove to hospital immediately.

Epilepsy

This is a condition which results from a tendency towards brief disruptions in the normal electrical activity of the brain. Epileptic fits may vary from momentary inattention without loss of consciousness (Minor Epilepsy) to muscular spasm and convulsions (Major Epilepsy).

People who are liable to epileptic fits generally carry an orange identification card or wear a warning bracelet.

MINOR EPILEPSY

This may start in childhood and may persist into adulthood. This type of fit can pass unnoticed because the casualty often only appears to be daydreaming.

Symptoms and Signs
- Casualty may appear to be in a daydream and be staring ahead blankly.
- Casualty might start behaving strangely; these "automatisms" include chewing or smacking lips, saying odd things, or fiddling with clothing.
- Casualty may have lost memory.

Aim
Keep calm and protect the casualty while consciousness is impaired. For example, prevent the casualty wandering on to a busy road.

Treatment
1 Do nothing except:

- Protect the person from any dangers such as busy roads.
- Keep other people away.
- Talk to the casualty quietly.

2 Stay with the casualty until you are certain that the person has recovered and can get home.

NB It is not unusual for a major fit to follow a minor one.

3 Advise the casualty to see a doctor.

MAJOR EPILEPSY

Most major epileptic attacks come on unexpectedly. However, sometimes a person experiences an *aura* which serves as a warning that something more severe is about to happen. The aura may differ from one person to another. For example, it may take the form of a strange feeling in the body or a particular smell or taste. During an aura a person's normal mood may be altered although this will not last long.

Symptoms and Signs

All cases of Major Epilepsy follow a two-stage pattern: rigidity/loss of consciousness followed by jerking.

● Casualty suddenly loses consciousness and falls to the ground, sometimes letting out a strange cry.

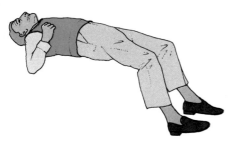

● The casualty becomes rigid for a few seconds and breathing may cease. Mouth and lips will turn blue (cyanosis) and there will be congestion about the face and in the neck.
● The muscles then relax and begin convulsive movements. They consist of contraction and relaxation of alternate groups of muscles. These convulsions may be quite vigorous.

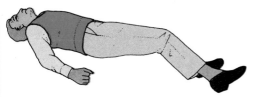

During this stage the breathing may become difficult or noisy through the clenched jaw; froth may appear around the mouth, blood stained if lips or tongue have been bitten; and there may be loss of control of the bladder and occasionally the bowel.

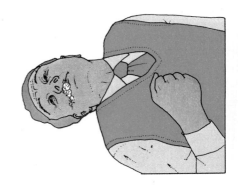

● Finally, the muscles will relax although the casualty will remain unconscious for a few minutes or more.

After the fit is over, usually five minutes at the most, breathing will return to normal and the casualty will regain consciousness but may feel dazed and confused and may act strangely. This feeling can last from several minutes to an hour and the person may want to rest quietly.

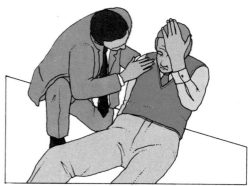

Aim
Protect the casualty from injury during the fit and provide care once consciousness is regained.

Treatment
1 If the casualty is falling, try to support or ease the fall and lay down gently.

2 Clear a space around the casualty and, unless you want someone to help, ask all bystanders to leave. If possible, carefully loosen clothing around the neck and place something soft under the head.

Do Not move or lift the casualty unless in danger.

Do Not forcibly restrain the casualty.

Do Not put anything in the casualty's mouth or try to open it.

3 When the convulsions cease, place the casualty in the Recovery Position to aid breathing (see p. 24).

Do Not try and wake the casualty.

4 When the attack is over stay with the casualty until you are certain recovery is complete.

Do Not give the casualty anything to drink until you are sure of full alertness.

5 Even if the casualty makes a full, quick recovery, advise the casualty to inform doctor about the latest attack.

Do Not send for an ambulance unless the casualty has several fits, has been injured during the fit or takes longer than fifteen minutes to regain consciousness. The epilepsy card may tell you how long the casualty normally takes to wake up.

Infantile Convulsions

In children between the ages of one and four, a raised temperature caused by the onset of an infectious disease or a throat or ear infection can cause convulsions. Despite their alarming nature, they are rarely dangerous but the symptoms may persist while the child's temperature remains abnormally high.

Symptoms and Signs
- Child has high fever and will be "flushed" and sweating.
- Twitching of muscles of face and limbs.
- Occasional squinting or upturned eyes.
- There may be stiffness or rigidity, with the head back and spine arched.
- Casualty may be holding breath.
- Congestion of the face and neck.
- Froth may appear at the mouth.

Aim
Protect the child from injury and cool to reduce the intensity of the fit. Seek medical aid and reassure the parents.

Treatment
1 Ensure a good supply of fresh air.

2 Loosen any constricting clothing around neck and chest.

3 Clear a space around the child if convulsions are severe.

4 Carry out the general treatment for the unconscious casualty.

5 Cool the child: first remove any covering bedclothes and/or clothes, then sponge with tepid water, starting from the head and working down.

Do Not allow the child to become too chilled.

6 Reassure the casualty's parents and advise them to call a doctor.

Hysteria

This is usually caused by an over-reaction to an emotional upset or nervous stress and is likely to be heightened by the presence of onlookers.

Symptoms and Signs
● Temporary loss of behavioural control with dramatic shouting, screaming, crying, wild beating of limbs. Casualty may be rolling around on the ground and/or tearing at hair and clothes.
● Hysterical over-breathing (hyperventilation) may follow.
● Casualty may be unable to move or be walking strangely for no apparent reason.

Aim
Isolate the casualty from any onlookers and gently but firmly help casualty to calm down enough to regain control.

Treatment
1 Reassure the casualty, refrain from showing any sympathy and, gently but firmly, escort to a quiet place.

Do Not physically restrain or slap the casualty; this may make the casualty more violent.

2 Stay with the casualty and keep under observation until fully recovered.

3 Advise the casualty to see a doctor.

Emergencies in Diabetes

Diabetes (diabetes mellitus) is a condition which arises when there is a disturbance in the way the body regulates the sugar concentrations in the blood. This can result in two conditions: too much sugar in the blood (hyperglycaemia) or too little sugar in the blood (hypoglycaemia). If prolonged, both conditions can result in unconsciousness and eventually, the death of a casualty. However, hyperglycaemia normally develops very gradually so it is rare for a First Aider to find a casualty in this condition.

Diabetics need to control their blood sugar levels carefully by balancing the amount of sugar in their diets with insulin injections or tablets. Most diabetics, including children, give their own treatments two or three times a day, and eat an appropriate amount of the correct types of food. As a result many carry hypodermic needles, insulin bottles or other medication on them all the time. Most diabetics will also carry a card or wear a bracelet (see p. 41) indicating that they have diabetes.

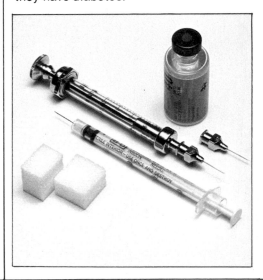

LOW BLOOD SUGAR (HYPOGLYCAEMIA)

If a diabetic has taken too much insulin by mistake, has eaten too little food or missed a meal or if exercise has burned up the sugar, the concentration of sugar in the blood falls. Low blood sugar will affect the brain and if prolonged or very low it will result in unconsciousness and the possible death of the casualty.

Symptoms and Signs
● A diabetic may feel faint, dizzy and light-headed and may be aware that sugar-level is low.
● Casualty might be confused and disorientated and may appear to be drunk and possibly aggressive.
● Skin becomes pale with profuse sweating.
● Pulse becomes rapid.
● Breathing becomes shallow and breath will be odourless.
● Limbs may begin to tremble.
● Casualty's level of responsiveness may deteriorate rapidly.

NB The longer a diabetic has been on insulin the less evident the early warning symptoms may become.

Aim
Restore the sugar/insulin balance as soon as possible. If the casualty is unconscious, arrange removal to hospital immediately.

Treatment

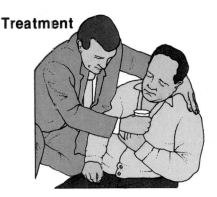

1 If the casualty is conscious and capable of swallowing, immediately give sugar lumps, a sugary drink, chocolate or other sweet food in order to raise the level of sugar in the blood.

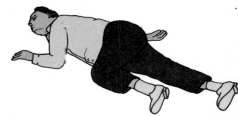

2 If the casualty is unconscious but breathing normally, place in the Recovery Position (see p. 24) and carry out the general treatment for the unconscious casualty.

3 Remove to hospital immediately.

Useful sugary foods
Very sweet tea
   or other sugary drink
Fruit juice
Sugar lumps
Cakes
Biscuits
Chocolate

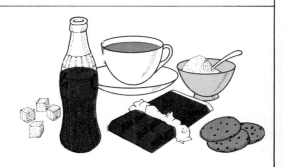

FRACTURES

A fracture is a broken or cracked bone. Although the outside of a bone is hard, it may crack or break if struck, twisted or overstressed. Generally, considerable force is required to break a bone. However, the elderly often have brittle bones and only slight force is needed to produce a break. Conversely, the long bones of infants can bend slightly.

All fractures must be handled very carefully; mishandling by the unskilled may result in further damage to the surrounding tissues.

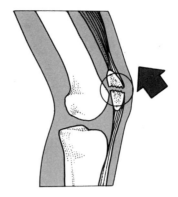

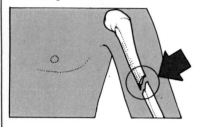

A bone can be fractured directly at the point where the force of a blow is applied. For example, if someone is struck by a moving vehicle the lower leg may be broken at the point where it was hit by the vehicle's bumper.

Another form of indirect force occurs when sudden, powerful, muscular contractions pull pieces of bone away from the point where the muscle is attached. For example, a footballer who tries to kick a ball but misses and hits the ground, can cause the knee-cap to snap in two because the powerful thigh muscles jerk suddenly at the anchorage points on that bone.

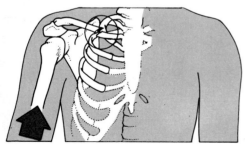

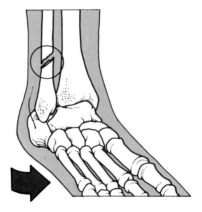

However, a bone can also be fractured indirectly at some distance from the spot where the force is applied. In this case, the bone is broken by the force being transmitted along it, or the adjacent bone, from the point of impact. For example, a fall on the outstretched hand may result in a fractured collar-bone.

In the same way, the "wrenching" of a joint can cause its ligaments to pull so hard at the joint that they fracture one of the bones to which they are attached. For example, a person who turns the foot over by tripping or stumbling may fracture a lower leg bone at the ankle.

THE SKELETON

The body is built on a framework of bones called the skeleton. This skeleton supports the body, gives it its basic shape and provides protection for the internal organs of the body. For example, the skull surrounds and protects the brain and the rib-cage protects the lungs, heart and other vital organs. The bones are also important for movement. They provide anchorage points for the muscles, and many of them also act as levers for the muscles to pull against.

Bones have blood vessels running through and alongside them. A fracture can result in severe blood loss mainly because of the damage to the surrounding tissues caused by the broken bone ends.

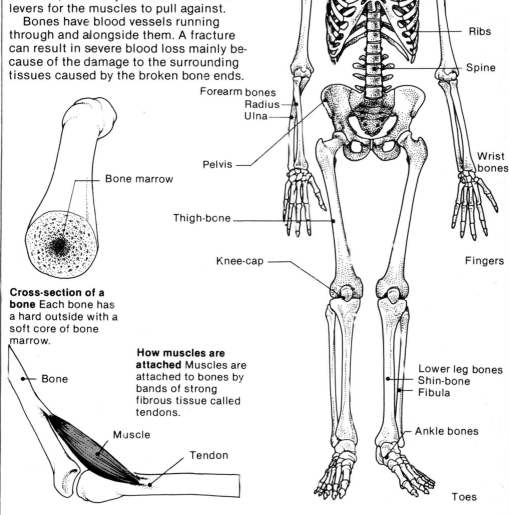

Skull

Upper arm bone

Jaw

Breastbone

Collar-bone

Shoulder-blade

Ribs

Spine

Forearm bones
Radius
Ulna

Pelvis

Wrist bones

Bone marrow

Thigh-bone

Fingers

Knee-cap

Cross-section of a bone Each bone has a hard outside with a soft core of bone marrow.

Bone

How muscles are attached Muscles are attached to bones by bands of strong fibrous tissue called tendons.

Lower leg bones
Shin-bone
Fibula

Muscle

Tendon

Ankle bones

Toes

Types of Fracture

Fractures fall into two categories, closed or open, and both can be complicated.

Closed Fracture
This is a fracture where the skin surface around the damaged bone is not broken.

Open Fracture
When a wound leads from the surface of the skin to the fracture or a broken bone end penetrates the surface of the skin, the fracture is said to be "open".

Open fractures are serious not only because they can result in severe external blood loss but also because germs can gain access to the soft tissues and the broken bone. Such infection can be dangerous and difficult to cure.

Complicated Fracture
Closed or open fractures are said to be "complicated" when there is an associated injury. For example, if an important structure, nerve or organ is damaged by the broken bone end or when a fracture is associated with a dislocated joint.

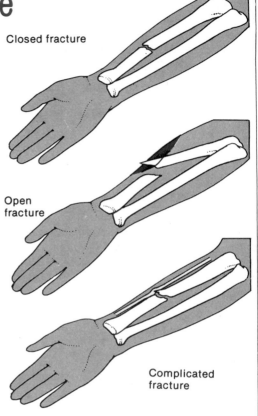

Closed fracture

Open fracture

Complicated fracture

General Symptoms and Signs
● The snap of the bone may have been felt or heard by the casualty.
● Pain at or near the site of injury increased by movement.
● Casualty may find it difficult or impossible to move the part normally.
● Tenderness at the site of the fracture when gentle pressure is applied over the affected area.
● Swelling and, later, bruising of the injured part. This may not be evident at first but will develop as blood leaks into the tissues; it may mask the true nature of the injury.
● Deformity at the site of the fracture. This may be irregularity of the bone; shortening, angulation or rotation of the

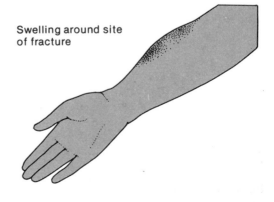

Swelling around site of fracture

limb (e.g., the limb has twisted further than is normally possible — a turned out foot is common with a fractured neck of thigh-bone), or depression of a flat bone.

● Coarse bony grating (crepitus) may be heard or felt upon examination — this should *never* be sought deliberately.

● Symptoms and signs of shock (see p. 90). The degree of shock will be particularly noticeable in those with a fractured thigh-bone or pelvis.

NB Not all the symptoms and signs will be present in every fracture. As many as possible should be noted by simple observation without moving any part unnecessarily. Compare the shape of the injured and uninjured limbs whenever possible. If you are in any doubt about the severity of an injury, treat as a fracture.

Aim

The keynote of First Aid treatment for any fracture is prevention of movement at the site of injury (immobilisation). Movement can not only make a fracture more painful but it frequently makes it worse. In all cases, arrange removal to hospital.

General Treatment

Casualties with fractures should *not* be moved unless it is absolutely necessary. Make the casualty as comfortable as possible, steady the part by hand or with padding and await the arrival of skilled help. If you must move the casualty do so carefully and gently to avoid further injury and increased pain.

Specific fractures are dealt with individually later in the chapter. However, the general rules for treatment of any fracture are as follows:

1 Difficulty in breathing, severe bleeding and unconsciousness must be dealt with *before* the fracture.

2 Treat all fractures in the position in which the casualty is found unless there is immediate danger to life or the casualty is exposed to bad weather.

If time will allow, temporarily immobilise and support a fractured limb before moving the casualty to safety.

3 Steady and support the injured limb by hand.

Do Not move the injured part unnecessarily.

4 *If removal to hospital is imminent*, gently support the injured part by hand. Place the casualty in the most comfortable position and support with rolled-up blankets or similar materials.

5 *If transportation to hospital will be delayed by more than 30 minutes but the journey will be short and smooth*, immobilise the injured part by securing it to a sound part of the body with padding and bandages.

NB Bandages should be firm enough to prevent movement but not so tight as to interfere with the circulation (see p. 178) or cause pain.

6 Raise the injured part after immobilising it to minimise discomfort and swelling.

7 *If the journey to hospital will be long — in excess of 30 minutes — and/or rough*, extra bandages and splints may be required.

8 To minimise shock, treat as on p. 90.

NB A fractured limb may be so deformed that it will be impossible to apply bandages or splints without some re-alignment of the limb. In this case carefully and gently apply traction to the end of the limb and straighten it as far as the casualty will allow causing as little pain as possible.

Open Fractures

IF THE BONE IS PROTRUDING FROM THE WOUND

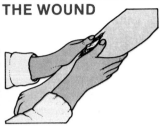

1 Control bleeding by applying pressure alongside the bone.

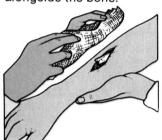

2 Gently place a piece of gauze over the protruding bone.

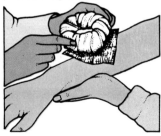

3 Place a ring pad or crescent-shaped pads of cotton wool or similar material around the wound. Build up padding around the bone until it is high enough to prevent pressure on the protruding bone.

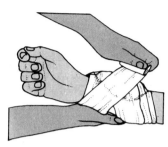

4 Secure dressings and pads with a bandage applied diagonally (see p. 187).

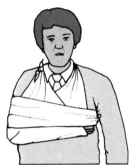

5 Elevate the injured part if possible and immobilise it.

6 Remove the casualty to hospital maintaining the treatment position. Transport as a stretcher case if necessary.

IF THERE IS NO BONE PROTRUDING FROM THE WOUND

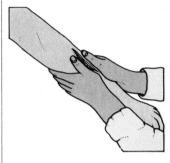

1 Control bleeding by squeezing the sides of the wound together gently but firmly.

Do Not apply firm downward pressure on the wound over the site of the fracture.

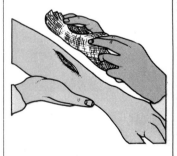

2 Place a dressing over the wound and pads of cotton wool around the edge of the wound.

3 Treat as in steps 4 – 6, left.

Skull Fractures

The skull provides a strong, protective case for the brain. Although damage to the bone may not appear to be significant, a "depressed" fracture or leakage of blood from the site of fracture may exert pressure on the brain (see p. 101).

Skull fractures may result in damage or disturbance to the brain, consciousness may be clouded or lost (see p. 98) and symptoms of any other injury or condition may be masked. Therefore, all head injuries should be regarded as serious, even if there is no sign of a wound.

A fracture of the crown of the head (cranium) is usually caused by a direct blow to the skull or a fall on the head; the bone may be depressed. A fracture of the base of the skull is usually caused by an indirect force such as a fall on to the feet or a blow to the jaw.

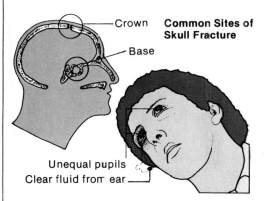

Crown — **Common Sites of Skull Fracture**

Base

Unequal pupils
Clear fluid from ear

Symptoms and Signs
- Obvious signs of head injury.
- Blood and/or clear, watery cerebrospinal fluid may issue from the ear or the nose.
- There may be a bloodshot and, later, a black eye.
- Pupils may be unequally dilated (see *Compression* p. 101).
- Brief or partial loss of consciousness.

Aim
Arrange urgent removal to hospital.

Treatment

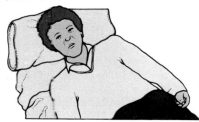

1 If the casualty is conscious, place in a half-sitting position with the head and shoulders supported.

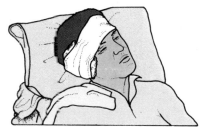

2 If any discharge issues from the ear, incline the head towards the injured side, cover the ear with a sterile dressing or similar pad and secure very lightly with bandage. *Do not* plug the ear.

3 If the casualty is unconscious but breathing normally, place in the Recovery Position (see p. 24) with the head lying on the affected side.

4 Check the breathing rate (see p. 12), pulse (see p. 89) and levels of responsiveness (see p. 98) at 10-minute intervals.

5 If breathing and heartbeat stop, begin resuscitation immediately (see pp. 18 – 21).

6 To minimise shock, treat as on p. 90.

7 Remove to hospital.

Jaw and Facial Fractures

Fractures and wounds to the jaw and face may be complicated by further damage to the brain, skull and/or bones in the neck. There are three serious risks associated with these injuries:

● The airway may be obstructed or blocked. This can be caused by: internal bleeding into the lungs and breathing passages (nose, mouth or throat); the tongue falling to the back of the throat if the casualty is unconscious; swollen, displaced or lacerated tissues in the throat; or broken or detached teeth.

● Inadequate or absent cough reflex which would allow secretions, blood and foreign matter to run unnoticed into the lungs, causing asphyxia.

● Possibility of severe bleeding. This may be profuse and alarming initially,

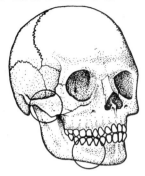

Common Fracture Sites of Face and Jaw

although it is not usually prolonged (see *Wounds and Bleeding*, pp. 78 – 81).

Injuries to the face may include the following: lower jaw fracture, cheek-bone and upper jaw fracture and nasal fracture.

LOWER JAW FRACTURE

This is usually the result of direct force, for example a heavy blow to the jaw. However, a blow to one side of the jaw can cause a fracture on the other side. Usually only one side of the jaw is affected but a fall on to the point of the chin can lead to a fracture of both sides of the jaw.

Symptoms and Signs

● Pain, increased by jaw movement or swallowing.

● Difficulty in speaking.

● The casualty feels nauseated.

● Casualty may dribble because of difficulty in swallowing. Saliva is normally stained by blood issuing from tooth sockets or other mouth wound.

● Wound inside the casualty's mouth.

● Swelling, tenderness and later bruising of the casualty's face and lower jaw.

● Irregularity may be felt along underside of jaw.

● Irregularity of the teeth may be seen.

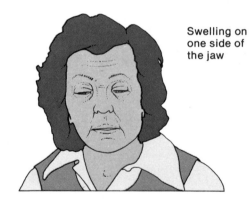

Swelling on one side of the jaw

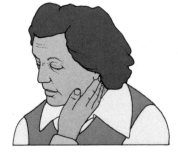

Irregularity may be felt along the jaw

Treatment

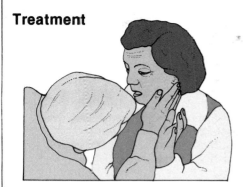

1 Maintain the casualty's breathing by ensuring a clear airway.

2 Control any bleeding and treat any wounds (see pp. 74 – 7).

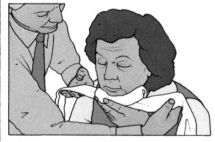

3 If conscious and not seriously injured, sit the casualty up with the head well-forward to allow any secretions to drain away.

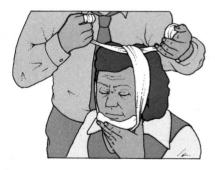

4 Support the jaw with a soft pad. Ask the casualty to hold it in place or, if necessary, tie a narrow bandage or other bandage around the casualty's head; tie the knot on the top of the head.

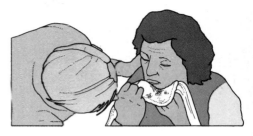

5 If vomiting occurs, quickly release the bandage and support the casualty's jaw and head. Gently clean out the casualty's mouth completely before replacing the bandage.

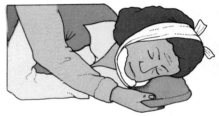

6 If the casualty is severely injured with downward displacement of the jaw or the casualty is, or becomes, unconscious and is breathing normally, place in the Recovery Position (see p. 24). Place a soft pad under the casualty's head to raise it and keep the weight off the jaw.

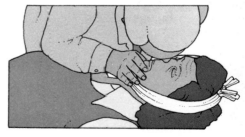

7 If breathing and heartbeat stop, begin resuscitation immediately (see pp. 18 – 21); you may need to use Mouth-to-Nose Ventilation.

8 Remove to hospital immediately maintaining the treatment position.

CHEEK-BONE AND UPPER JAW FRACTURE

Although there may not be any obvious signs of soft tissue wounds around the injury, there will probably be a significant amount of blood issuing from the nose. Severe swelling of the face and bruising around the eyes will develop rapidly; this may affect breathing. The casualty should be removed to hospital as soon as possible.

Treatment

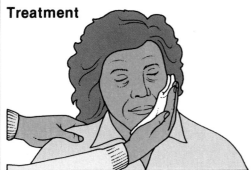

1 Place a cold compress (see p. 176) over the injured area to lessen swelling, bleeding and pain. Make sure you do not interfere with breathing and that bleeding from any mouth wound does not obstruct airway.

2 Treat any mouth wound (see p. 76).

3 Remove to hospital.

NASAL FRACTURE

Besides bleeding, the main problem associated with a nasal fracture is blockage of the airway so every effort must be made to ensure that the casualty has an open airway. A cold compress may provide some relief (see p. 176).

Usually there is no pressing need to immobilise a nasal fracture. Treat any nose-bleed (see p. 75) and remove the casualty to hospital.

THE SPINE

Made up of a series of small bones or "vertebrae", the spine forms a canal through which the spinal cord, runs (see p. 97). Almost all vertebrae are separated by a pad of cartilage called an inter-vertebral disc. The vertebrae have limited movement upon these discs, which act as a form of "shock-absorber" in case the spinal column is jarred. The whole column of bones is supported by numerous strong ligaments and the muscles of the trunk.

The spinal cord consists of nerve fibres which run from the brain and control many of the functions of the body. It is very delicate, and damage to it can result in loss of power or sensation in all parts of the body *below* the injured area. Temporary damage can occur if the cord is pinched by dislocated discs or bone fragments; permanent damage will

Spine Fractures

A fractured spine is always classed as a serious injury, necessitating the greatest care in handling because it may be complicated by damage to the spinal cord.

Injury can result from both direct and indirect force. Impact from vehicle collisions and from heavy objects falling across the casualty's back, or severe jarring of the spine by falling on to the feet, buttocks or head can all result in serious spine injury.

"Whiplash" results from the violent backward movement of a person's head which commonly occurs when a vehicle is run into from behind. With this type of injury there may be severe muscular damage or, occasionally, the neck may be broken.

The two most vulnerable areas of the spinal column are the bones in the neck and the lower back.

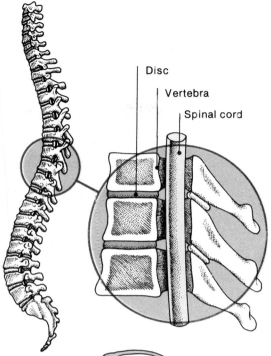

Disc

Vertebra

Spinal cord

occur if the cord is partially or completely severed.

Possible injuries to the spine include fractures, displaced intervertebral discs, strains and sprains; fractures may involve nerve damage. Slipped discs, strains and sprains are dealt with in the chapter on *Injuries to Muscles, Ligaments and Joints*, (see pp. 128 – 33). However, if you have any doubt about the nature of the injury it *must* be treated as a fracture. Always suspect a fracture if the casualty has a history of spine injury.

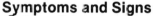

Symptoms and Signs

● Casualty may complain of severe pain in the back and may feel "cut in half".
● Casualty may have no control over limbs; ask the casualty to move wrists, ankles, fingers and toes.
● Possible loss of sensation. Test this by gently touching limbs without the casualty's knowledge and ask if anything can be felt.
● Irregularity may be felt on gentle examination.

Aim

Direct impact

Jarring

Prevent any further damage by immobilising the spine. Avoid moving the casualty unless absolutely necessary and arrange removal to hospital as soon as possible.

Treatment

FOR A FRACTURED BACK

1 Advise the casualty not to try to move.

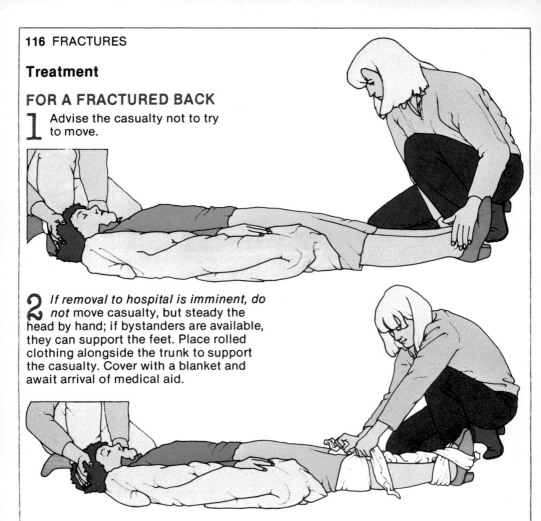

2 *If removal to hospital is imminent, do not* move casualty, but steady the head by hand; if bystanders are available, they can support the feet. Place rolled clothing alongside the trunk to support the casualty. Cover with a blanket and await arrival of medical aid.

3 *If removal to hospital will be delayed or the journey will be long and/or rough*, support the casualty's shoulders and pelvis and carefully place soft padding between the lower limbs. Tie a figure-of-eight bandage around the ankles and feet and broad bandages around the thighs and knees.

4 Remove to hospital. Transport the casualty on a rigid stretcher in the position found maintaining an open airway throughout.

FOR A FRACTURED NECK

1 Advise the casualty not to move. Support the head and neck until skilled help arrives.

2 *If removal to hospital will be delayed*, loosen clothing at neck and fit a neck collar as shown opposite.

3 Cover casualty with a blanket and await the arrival of the ambulance.

4 *If the casualty must be moved*, follow the procedure described for a fractured back, above.

FITTING A NECK (CERVICAL) COLLAR

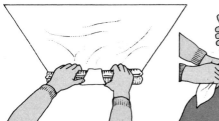

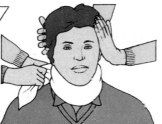

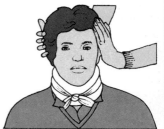

1 If a cervical collar is not available, fold a newspaper to a width of about 10 cm (4 in).

2 Wrap it in a triangular bandage or insert it into a stocking or leg of a pair of tights.

3 Place the centre of the collar at the front of the casualty's neck below the chin.

4 Fold the collar around the casualty's neck and tie in position at the front of the neck.

5 Ensure there is no obstruction to breathing.

UPPER TRUNK AND LIMBS

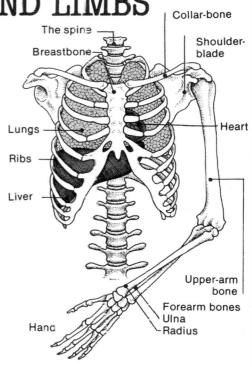

The *ribs* consist of 12 pairs of curved bones which extend from the vertebrae round to the front of the body.

The *chest cavity* is bounded in front by the breastbone, behind by the spine, below by the diaphragm, then encircled by the ribs. It contains the heart and major blood vessels, the lungs and the gullet.

The *shoulder girdle* and *upper limbs* consist of the collar-bone, the shoulder-blade (which is rarely broken) and the arm bones. The *collar-bone* is situated between the upper part of the breastbone and the shoulder, and forms a strut to hold the upper limbs away from the chest and support the neck and head. The *shoulder-blade* forms a joint with the collar-bone and the *upper-arm bone.*

Each upper limb consists of the upper-arm bone; the two bones in the forearm which allow for the turning action of the wrist; and the small bones at the wrist.

More bones form the framework of the palm of the hand and there are several small bones in the fingers and thumb.

Labels on diagram: The spine · Breastbone · Collar-bone · Shoulder-blade · Lungs · Heart · Ribs · Liver · Upper-arm bone · Forearm bones · Ulna · Radius · Hand

Rib and Breastbone Fractures

Rib fractures usually result from direct force, such as a blow to, or heavy fall on to, the chest, or from indirect force as a result of being crushed. If the fracture is complicated by a "sucking wound" of the chest (see p. 79) or by "paradoxical breathing" due to a stove-in-chest (see p. 57), asphyxia may result unless the injuries are treated immediately.

Symptoms and Signs
● General symptoms and signs of fracture.
● Casualty may feel a sharp pain at the site of the fracture, increased by anything more than shallow breathing or by coughing.
● Possible symptoms and signs of internal bleeding (see pp. 70 – 2) indicating damage to internal organs such as the lungs or liver.
● There may be an open wound of the chest wall over the fracture causing a "sucking wound" of the chest.
● Possible paradoxical breathing if there are multiple fractures (see p. 57).

Aim
Immobilise fracture and arrange removal to hospital.

Treatment

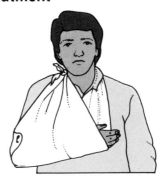

1 Support the limb on the injured side in an arm sling (see p. 181).

2 Remove to hospital. Transport as a sitting or walking casualty unless there are complications.

FOR A COMPLICATED FRACTURE
1 Immediately treat any "sucking" wound (see p. 79).

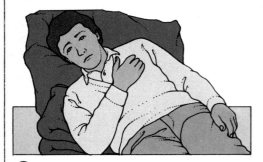

2 Lay the casualty down in a half-sitting position with the head and shoulders supported and the body inclined towards the injured side. Support the casualty by placing a folded blanket lengthwise along the back.

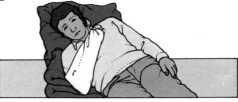

3 Support the limb on the injured side in an elevation sling (see p. 182).

4 If the casualty is unconscious or breathing becomes difficult and/or noisy, place in the Recovery Position (see p. 24) with the uninjured side uppermost.

5 Remove to hospital. Transport as a stretcher case maintaining the treatment position.

Collar-bone Fractures

A collar-bone fracture is commonly caused by indirect force resulting from a fall on to an outstretched hand or the point of the shoulder. Collar-bone fractures due to direct force are rare.

Symptoms and Signs
● General symptoms and signs of fracture.
● Pain and tenderness at the site of injury increased by movement.

● Casualty is reluctant to move the limb on the injured side.
● Casualty may support the arm on the injured side at the elbow and may keep the head inclined towards the injured side to relieve pain.
● Swelling or deformity may be seen or felt over the site of fracture.

Aim
Remove casualty to hospital.

Treatment

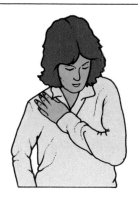

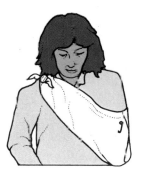

1 Gently place the limb on the injured side across the casualty's chest with the fingertips almost resting on the opposite shoulder.

3 Support the limb and padding in an elevation sling (see p. 182).

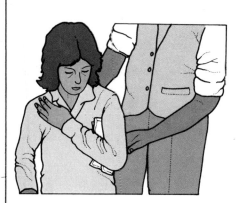

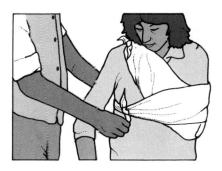

2 Place padding between the limb and chest on the affected side.

4 For additional support, secure the limb to the chest by applying a broad bandage over the sling; tie the knot in front on the uninjured side.

5 Remove to hospital.

Arm Fractures

Fractures can occur anywhere along the length of the upper-arm bone or the two forearm bones, and may involve the elbow. The bones most frequently broken, however, are those at the wrist (Colles fracture).

Fractures involving the elbow joint are especially common in children. This fracture may cause extensive damage to the surrounding blood vessels and nerves.

Symptoms and Signs
● General symptoms and signs of fracture.
● Pain at the site of fracture increased by movement.
● Casualty is unable to use the injured arm.
● Inability to bend the elbow if the joint is involved.

Aim
Remove to hospital.

Treatment

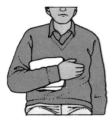

1 Gently support the injured limb across the casualty's chest. Place soft padding between the injured limb and the chest.

If wrist or forearm is injured, place in an extra fold of soft padding.

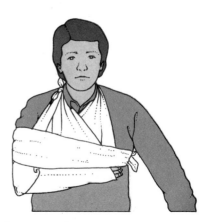

3 For additional support, secure the limb to the chest with a broad bandage applied over the sling; tie the knot in front on the uninjured side.

4 Remove to hospital.

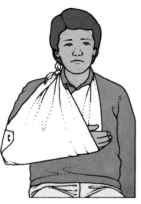

2 Support limb and padding in an arm sling (see p. 181).

IF THE ELBOW CANNOT BE BENT

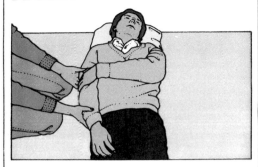

1 Lay the casualty down and place the injured limb by the side of the trunk. *Do not* attempt to bend the elbow forcibly. Ask the casualty to support it in that position with the other hand if possible. Place soft padding between the injured limb and the body.

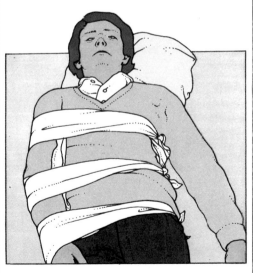

2 Secure the injured limb to the body by three broad bandages: around the wrist and thighs, around the upper arm and trunk, around the forearm and trunk.

3 Remove casualty to hospital. Transport as a stretcher case maintaining the treatment position.

Hand and Finger Fractures

Fractures of the hand are usually due to direct force. They are sometimes the result of crush injuries and may involve severe bleeding.

Symptoms and Signs
- General symptoms and signs of fracture.
- Casualty is unable to use fingers.
- Extensive swelling and bruising at the site of injury.

Aim
Immobilise the injured hand and remove the casualty to hospital.

Treatment
1 Control bleeding (see p. 28) and treat any wounds.

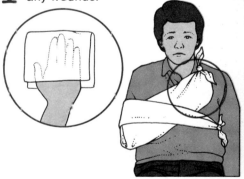

2 Protect the injured hand by placing in a fold of soft padding.

3 Gently support the affected limb in an elevation sling (see p. 182).

4 For additional support, secure the limb to the chest by applying a broad bandage over the sling; tie the knot in front on the uninjured side.

5 Remove to hospital.

LOWER TRUNK AND LIMBS

The *pelvis* is a basin-shaped structure of bone attached to the lower part of the spine. It supports and protects the contents of the lower abdominal cavity and contains sockets for the hip joints.

Each *lower limb* consists of: the thigh-bone; the two bones of the lower leg, the shin-bone (tibia) and the fibula; and a number of smaller bones in the foot and ankle. The thigh-bone reaches from the hip to the knee and is the longest and strongest bone in the body. At its lower end it forms part of the knee-joint, at its upper end its head fits into the pelvis.

The *knee-cap* is a small, flattish bone which lies in front of the knee-joint. The two bones in the lower leg extend from the knee to the ankle, the long thin bone (fibula) lies on the outer side of the thicker shin-bone.

There are several small bones which form the heel, instep (arch) and toes.

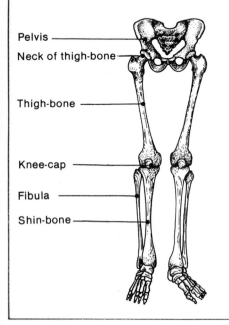

Pelvis
Neck of thigh-bone
Thigh-bone
Knee-cap
Fibula
Shin-bone

Pelvic Fractures

These are usually caused by a direct crush injury or by indirect force such as might occur during vehicle collisions. For example, the impact of a knee on a car's fascia can force the head of the femur through the socket of the hip-joint.

One or both sides of the pelvic girdle may be fractured and pelvic injuries can be complicated by injury to the bladder and urinary passages.

Symptoms and Signs
● General symptoms and signs of fracture.
● Pain and tenderness in the region of the hips and groin which is increased by movement.
● Casualty is unable to walk or even stand although the legs appear sound.
● Casualty may express a great desire to pass water if the bladder or urinary passages are damaged. If the casualty does pass water it may be bloodstained.
● Symptoms and signs of shock (see p. 90).

Aim
Make casualty comfortable and arrange urgent removal to hospital.

Treatment

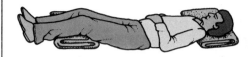

1 Place the casualty on the back with legs straight or, if it is more comfortable for the casualty, bend the knees slightly and place a rolled blanket underneath them.

2 If the casualty expresses a desire to pass water, advise against it; urine may escape into the tissues.

3 *If removal to hospital is imminent,* cover the casualty with a blanket and await the arrival of the ambulance.

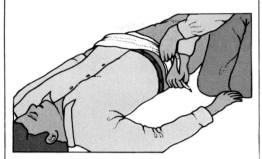

4 *If ambulance is delayed or the journey to hospital will be long — in excess of 30 minutes — and/or rough,* gently apply two broad bandages around the pelvis, the lower one first. Overlap them by half with the centres lined up with the hip joint on the injured side. Tie off on uninjured side. (If both sides of the pelvis are fractured, tie off in the centre.)

5 Place adequate soft padding between the knees and ankles.

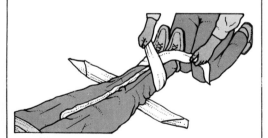

6 Apply a figure-of-eight bandage around the ankles and feet and a broad bandage around the knees. Tie knots on the uninjured side.

7 To minimise shock, treat as on p. 90.

8 Remove to hospital. Transport as a stretcher case, maintaining the treatment position.

Hip and Thigh-bone Fractures

A fracture can occur anywhere along the length of the thigh-bone. It is the longest bone in the body and has a rich blood supply. All incidents where the thigh-bone is fractured should be regarded as serious because, in most cases, a large volume of blood is lost into the tissues and this may result in severe shock (see p. 90).

This type of fracture often results from falls and road traffic accidents. In the aged a fracture may result from a minor fall; in most adults, however, considerable force is required to break the femur.

Fractures of the hip-joint involving the neck or upper portion of the thigh-bone are often mistaken for a badly bruised hip. Any elderly person who complains of pain in the hip after a fall or other minor accident should be considered as having a possible neck of femur fracture and removed to hospital.

Symptoms and Signs
● General symptoms and signs of fracture.
● Visible deformity in lower limb: if fracture of the shaft, the limb may be shortened by contraction of muscles around fractured bone; if fracture of the neck, the foot may be turned outwards.
● Symptoms and signs of shock (see p. 90).

Treatment
See Treatment for Lower Limb Fracture, over.

Leg Fractures

Either or both of the two bones of the lower leg, the shin-bone (tibia) and the fibula, may be broken. Fractures of the upper end of the shin-bone commonly occur when pedestrians are hit by car bumpers and are known as "bumper" fractures. Shin-bone fractures are often open because only a thin layer of skin and tissue covers the bone.

The fibula is most commonly broken by "wrenching" of the ankle joint. However, because this is not a weight-bearing bone, a simple fracture is often mistaken for a severe sprain, especially if a crack fracture occurs a few inches above the ankle. As a result, the casualty may not seek medical advice until a few days after the injury.

Common Sites of Leg Fracture

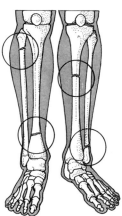

Symptoms and Signs
● General symptoms and signs of fracture.
● Swelling and bruising apparent.
● Angulation and rotation will be seen only if both bones are broken.
● Deformity may be seen or felt along one or both bones.
● Possible "open" wound if shin-bone fractured.
● Possible symptoms and signs of shock (see p. 90).

Treatment for Lower Limb Fracture

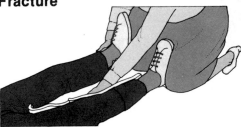

1 Lay the casualty down and carefully steady and support the limb by hand.

2 *If the journey to hospital will be short (i.e., less than 30 minutes) and smooth*, place bandages in position under the feet and knees.

3 Place plenty of soft padding between the knees and ankles.

4 Gently bring the sound limb alongside the injured limb.

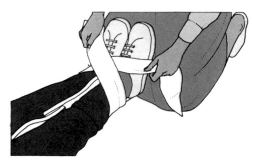

5 Tie a figure-of-eight bandage around the feet and ankles and a broad bandage around the knees; tie all the knots on the uninjured side.

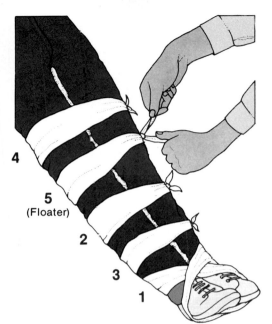

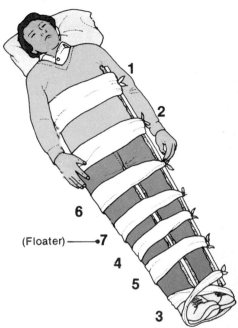

6 *If the journey to hospital will be long and/or rough and there are no splints available*, apply additional padding and three more bandages: one around the lower legs, one around the thighs, and finally one "floater" bandage below the fracture site; avoid the fracture site.

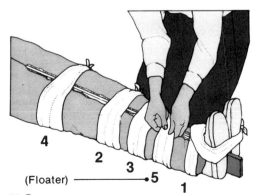

If *splints are available* (for a fractured leg) support the injured limb and place a splint with adequate padding between the legs extending from crotch to foot. Apply padding and bandage as for a rough journey, above.

If *the thigh-bone is fractured*, place an additional longer splint and padding along the outside of the fractured limb extending from armpit to foot.

Apply additional padding on the outside of the limb where the splint touches bony areas, at the ankles and hips for example, and in any hollows.

Secure the top end of the long splint with two broad bandages: one around the chest just below the armpits and one around the pelvis in line with the hip joints. Then bandage the lower legs and splints as for a rough journey, see left. Tie knots over the splint.

7 To minimise shock, treat as on p. 90.

8 When the limbs are immobilised, raise them slightly to minimise discomfort and swelling.

9 Remove to hospital: transport as a stretcher case maintaining the treatment position.

Knee-cap Fractures

This small bone lies in front of the knee joint and forms the anchorage point for the large muscles of the thigh and the ligaments from the shin-bone. It may be fractured by a direct blow or as the result of muscular action, such as a mis-kick.

Symptoms and Signs
- General symptoms and signs of fracture.
- Severe pain at knee, mainly at front.
- Tenderness around the knee-cap.
- Loss of movement of knee-joint; casualty is unable to bend the knee.
- Considerable swelling and, later, bruising may be present.

Treatment

1 Lay the casualty on the back with the head and shoulders raised and supported with rolled blankets or coats.

2 Gently raise and support the injured limb on a splint extending from the buttocks to beyond the heel which is covered with adequate padding. Apply extra padding under the knee, but only sufficient to fill the hollow. Place adequate padding under the heel in order to raise it off the splint.

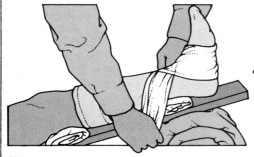

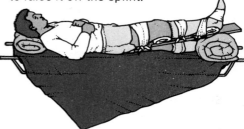

3 Apply a figure-of-eight bandage around the ankle, foot and splint; tie the knots against the side of the splint. Apply broad bandages around the thigh and splint and around the lower leg and splint. Tie off on the outer side of the fractured limb.

4 Remove to hospital; transport as a stretcher case maintaining the treatment position.

Foot Fractures

Fractures of the foot often result from direct injuries such as being run over or hit or crushed by heavy objects. However, injury can also result from twisting falls or jumps.

Symptoms and Signs
- General symptoms and signs of fracture.
- Pain in foot increased by movement.
- Tenderness at fracture site.
- Loss of movement of foot; casualty unable to walk properly on foot.
- Swelling and bruising may be present at site of injury.
- Deformity, such as irregularity of the bony arch may be present.

Treatment

1 Lay the casualty down.

2 Raise and support the injured foot.

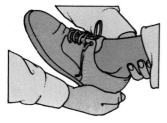 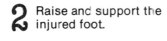 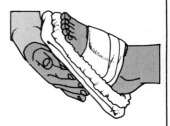

3 Gently remove the shoe and sock (see p. 44).

4 Control bleeding and dress any wounds.

5 Place a splint with adequate padding on the sole of the foot.

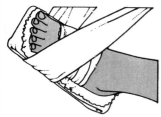 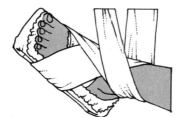 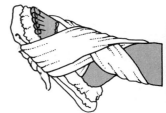

6 Secure with a figure-of-eight bandage. Place centre of broad bandage over splint on sole of foot and cross the ends over the instep.

7 Take ends around behind ankle, cross them again and bring them around to the front.

8 Cross them once more over the instep and take them under the foot; tie off over splint.

9 Keep the foot raised and supported.

10 Remove to hospital; transport as a stretcher case, maintaining the treatment position.

INJURIES TO MUSCLES, LIGAMENTS AND JOINTS

Injuries which involve damage to the muscles, joints or ligaments which strengthen the joints are common and they can be painful.

A dislocated joint in particular may also be mistaken for, or accompanied by, a fracture. In all cases where you are in doubt about the injury, treat the injury as a fracture and arrange for removal to hospital as soon as possible.

THE MUSCLES

These cause the various parts of the body to move and are of two types: voluntary and involuntary; both produce movement by contracting and relaxing.

Voluntary muscles are so-called because they are under the control of the will. Their movement is co-ordinated through the motor nerves which pass directly from the brain or via the spinal cord (see p. 97). The bones of the skeleton act as a framework for these muscles to pull against and the muscles are attached to the bones by bands of strong, fibrous tissue called *tendons*. Voluntary muscles operate in pairs: one muscle or group of muscles contracts in order to move a bone at the same time as its paired muscle or group of muscles relaxes so that movement can take place.

Involuntary muscles operate the vital organs, such as the heart and intestines, and work all the time, even when we sleep. Most of these muscles cannot be controlled by the will but only by the nerves in the autonomic nervous system (see p. 97).

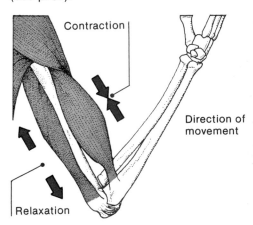

Contraction

Direction of movement

Relaxation

THE JOINTS

Joints are formed by the junction of two or more bones and there are two types: immovable and movable.

Immovable joints are those where the bone edges fit firmly into each other or are fused together so that no movement can take place. The best example of this type of joint is in the skull.

Movable joints can either allow free movement in all directions (ball-and-socket joints), movement in one plane only (hinge joints) or only limited movement (slightly movable joints).

The ends of any bones forming a joint are covered in a smooth cartilage to minimise friction and the joint is strengthened by bands of strong tissue called *ligaments*. The joint itself is enclosed in a capsule filled with a lubricant called synovial fluid.

BALL-AND-SOCKET JOINTS

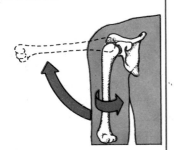

Formed by the round head of one bone fitting into the cup-shaped cavity of another, ball-and-socket joints allow movement in all directions. Examples are the shoulder and hip joints.

HINGE JOINTS

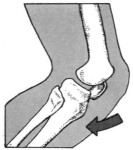

When the surfaces of the bones are moulded together they only allow movement in one direction — bending (flexion) and straightening (extension). Examples are the elbow and knee joints.

SLIGHTLY MOVABLE JOINTS

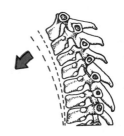

With this type of joint only limited movement is possible. Examples are the joints between the vertebrae and those between the ribs and the spine.

Strain

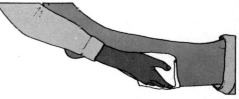

A strain occurs when a muscle or group of muscles is over-stretched and possibly torn, by violent or sudden movement. This might occur when a person is lifting heavy weights incorrectly or participating in sports.

Symptoms and Signs

- Sudden, sharp pain at the site of the injury which may radiate outwards with subsequent stiffness and/or cramp.
- Swelling at the site of injury.

Aim

Make the casualty as comfortable as possible and seek medical aid.

Treatment

1 Place the casualty in the most comfortable position.

2 Steady and support the injured part; elevate an injured limb.

3 Apply a cold compress if the strain is of recent origin (see p. 176).

4 If you are in any doubt about the casualty's condition, treat as a fracture (see pp. 106 – 127).

5 Remove to hospital.

FOR BACK STRAIN

If the casualty is in extreme pain and reluctant to move, lay the casualty down on a firm surface, place a cold compress on the back (see p. 176) and seek medical aid.

If you are in any doubt about the severity of the injury treat as a fractured spine (see p 114).

Sprain

This is an injury which occurs at a joint when the ligaments and tissues around that particular joint are suddenly "wrenched" or torn. For example, a sprained ankle may result if your foot turns over unexpectedly while walking or running. Some sprains are minor, others are associated with extensive damage to the tissues and are difficult to distinguish from fractures. In all doubtful cases, treat the injury as a fracture.

Symptoms and Signs
● Pain and tenderness around the joint increased by movement.
● Swelling around the joint followed later by bruising.

Aim
Make the casualty as comfortable as possible.

Treatment

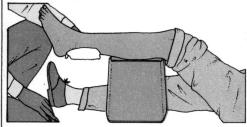

1 Rest and support the injured part in the most comfortable position for the casualty; elevate an injured limb.

2 Carefully expose the joint and, if sprain is of recent origin, apply a cold compress (see p. 176) to reduce swelling and pain.

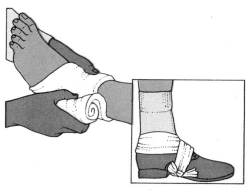

3 Alternatively, help counteract swelling and provide some support by surrounding the joint with a thick layer of cotton wool; secure with a bandage.

If an ankle is sprained where skilled help is not available *do not* remove the shoe or sock but apply a figure-of-eight bandage over the boot or shoe.

4 If the symptoms persist, seek medical aid.

If you are in doubt about the injury, treat as a fracture (see pp. 106 – 127).

Dislocation

This is the displacement of one or more bones at a joint. It occurs when a strong force acts directly or indirectly on a joint wrenching a bone into an abnormal position. Alternatively, it can be the result of a sudden muscular contraction.

Joints which are most frequently dislocated are the shoulder, elbow, thumb, finger and jaw. In some cases it is diffi-cult or even impossible to distinguish between a dislocation and a fracture and both may be present. If in doubt, *always* treat as a fracture.

Symptoms and Signs
● Casualty complains of severe (often sickening) pain at or near the joint.
● Casualty is unable to move affected

part: joint "fixed" in position.
- Injured joint appears deformed.
- Swelling and later bruising at the site of injury.

Aim
Make the casualty as comfortable as possible and arrange removal to hospital.

Treatment
1 Support the injured part in the most comfortable position for the casualty

using pillows or cushions. Immobilise with bandages or slings if available.

2 Remove to hospital immediately.

Do Not attempt to replace bones in their normal positions as further damage to surrounding tissues may result. If in any doubt about the casualty's injury treat as a fracture (see pp. 106 – 127).

Displaced Cartilage of the Knee (Locked Knee)

The knee-joint contains two separate semi-lunar cartilages one of which may become displaced or torn. This can be caused by a sporting incident, such as a missed kick, by slipping off a step or by twisting the body whilst the weight is balanced on one leg.

Aim
Make the casualty as comfortable as possible and arrange removal to hospital.

Symptoms and Signs
- Casualty complains of severe sickening pain around the knee, more commonly on the inner side.
- The injured knee is held in a bent position. Although it may be further flexed, it cannot be straightened.
- Swelling may occur due to fluid collecting in the joint.

Treatment
1 Support the injured leg in the most comfortable position for the casualty.

Do Not change the bent position of the knee or attempt to straighten it.

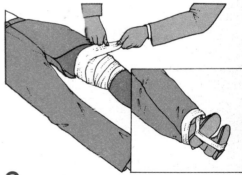

2 Protect the knee by placing soft padding around the joint; make sure that it extends well above and below the joint. Secure with a bandage; tie it firmly enough to support the knee but not so tight as to cause discomfort or affect circulation (see p. 178).

If necessary, immobilise the injured knee by crossing it over the sound leg and bandaging over the ankles. Alternatively, place padding such as a pillow under and around the leg.

3 Remove to hospital maintaining the treatment position.

Displaced Intervertebral Disc

Commonly known as a "slipped disc", this occurs when a piece of the cartilage which separates the bones in the spinal column protrudes backwards into the spinal cord. It can be a very painful condition although the onset of pain may be sudden or gradual.

Symptoms and Signs
● Severe, sharp pain in the back which may radiate towards the legs and may be increased by movement.

● Casualty may be unable or reluctant to move the neck or back.

Aim
Make casualty comfortable and seek medical aid.

Treatment
1 Lay the casualty down on a firm surface in the most comfortable position.

2 Seek medical aid.

Cramp

A cramp is a sudden, involuntary and painful contraction of a muscle or group of muscles. It can occur if there is poor muscular co-ordination during exercise; if chilling occurs following or during exercise such as swimming; if the body loses excessive amounts of salt and body fluids through severe sweating, diarrhoea or persistent vomiting; or during sleep. Cramps due to salt and water loss may also be associated with heat exhaustion (see p. 148).

This condition is normally relieved by stretching the muscles. First straighten the affected part of the body, then gently massage it.

Symptoms and Signs
● Pain in the affected area.
● Feeling of tightness or spasm in the affected muscles.
● Casualty is unable to relax contracted muscles.

Treatment
FOR CRAMP IN HAND
Gently, but firmly, straighten out the fingers and gently massage the area.

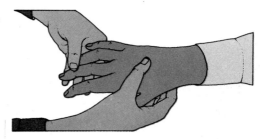

FOR CRAMP IN THIGH MUSCLES
Straighten the knee and raise the leg with one hand under the heel; with the other hand, press down the knee. Gently massage the affected muscles.

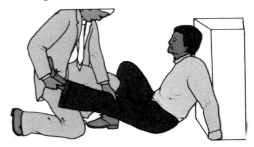

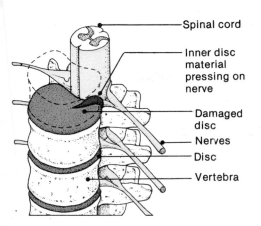

- Spinal cord
- Inner disc material pressing on nerve
- Damaged disc
- Nerves
- Disc
- Vertebra

FOR CRAMP IN CALF MUSCLES

Straighten the knee and gently draw the casualty's foot upwards towards the shin. Gently massage the affected muscles.

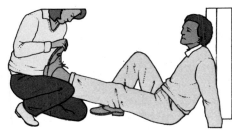

FOR CRAMP IN FOOT MUSCLES

Straighten out the casualty's toes and help the casualty to stand on the ball of the foot. Gently massage the foot.

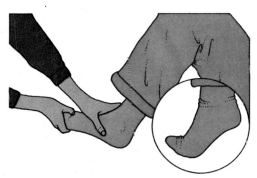

Hernia

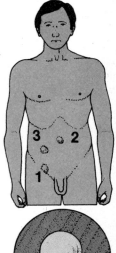

An abdominal hernia or rupture is a protrusion caused by a part of the contents of the abdomen protruding through the muscular wall under the skin.

A hernia occurs most frequently in the groin (1) but it is not uncommon at the navel (2) or through the scar of an abdominal operation (3). It may happen after exercise, while lifting heavy objects or when coughing.

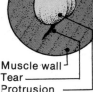

Muscle wall
Tear
Protrusion

Symptoms and Signs

● Painless swelling which may persist or worsen or there may be sudden, painful swelling with possible vomiting. (The latter may indicate a "strangulated" hernia which is a serious condition requiring urgent medical attention.)

Treatment

1 Reassure the casualty.

2 Lay the casualty down in a half-sitting position, support the head and shoulders. Bend the knees and support in this position.

3 If vomiting occurs, or seems likely, place the casualty in the Recovery Position (see p. 24).

4 Seek medical aid.

Do Not attempt to reduce the swelling.

BURNS AND SCALDS

These are injuries to body tissues caused by heat, chemicals or radiation. Burns caused by "wet" heat such as steam or hot liquids, are called scalds. Burns vary in depth, size and severity and may damage the underlying parts of the body as well as the skin. Most burns will require medical attention.

Heat is the most common cause of burns. Other causes include contact with dry or liquid corrosive chemicals whether acid or alkali, and over-exposure to radiation and sun rays.

There is considerable risk of infection with burns because, in damaging the skin, burns reduce the skin's protection against germs. There is also a danger of shock developing, because serum leaks out of the circulatory system into the burnt area (see p. 90).

Types of Burn

Dry Burns
Flames, lighted cigarettes and hot electrical equipment such as irons are all common causes of dry burns.

Fast-moving objects rubbed against the skin produce dry friction burns. Alternatively, they may be caused by the skin rubbing against an object. The most common example of this is a "rope burn".

Scalds
Wet heat such as steam, hot water or fat produces scalds.

Cold Burns
Contact with substances such as liquid oxygen and liquid nitrogen can cause cold burns.

Chemical Burns
Acids and alkalis, found in domestic cleaning products as well as in industry, may cause burns when they come into contact with the skin.

Electrical Burns
Electrical currents and lightning generate heat and burn skin and underlying tissues.

Radiation Burns
Sun rays and light reflected from bright surfaces, (e.g., snow) can damage the skin and eyes.

Very rarely, radiation burns can come from X-rays. An overdose is absorbed by the skin causing burns.

Classification of Burns

Burns are classified according to the area and depth of the injury. These factors will determine what treatment is required and whether the casualty needs hospital attention. However, any casualty with burns covering an area greater than 2.5 cm (1 in) square, involving more than the surface of the skin or burns arising from electrical contact, must be referred to a doctor or hospital.

AREA
The area of a burn gives a rough guide as to whether or not a casualty is likely to suffer shock. The greater the area involved, the greater the possibility of shock, because of greater fluid loss. For example, an otherwise fit adult casualty with a superficial burn covering 9% or more of the body's surface will need hospital treatment (see diagram opposite).

SEVERITY OF BURNS

There are three levels of burning: superficial, intermediate and deep or full-thickness burns. However, it is often difficult to distinguish between the different levels, particularly in the early stages. A large burn will almost certainly contain areas of all three.

Superficial Burns

These burns involve only the outer layers of skin and result in general redness, swelling and extreme tenderness. This type of burn usually heals well.

Intermediate Burns

These burns involve the formation of blisters and the area around the burn will be swollen and red. These burns can be infected so you should seek medical aid.

Deep Burns

These burns involve all layers of skin. The skin appears pale, waxy and sometimes, charred. These burns will be relatively pain-free because the nerves are damaged. Deep burns *always* require medical attention.

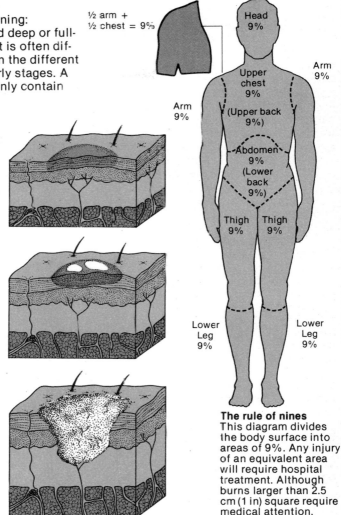

½ arm + ½ chest = 9%

Head 9%

Arm 9%

Upper chest 9%

(Upper back 9%)

Arm 9%

Abdomen 9% (Lower back 9%)

Thigh 9% Thigh 9%

Lower Leg 9% Lower Leg 9%

The rule of nines
This diagram divides the body surface into areas of 9%. Any injury of an equivalent area will require hospital treatment. Although burns larger than 2.5 cm (1 in) square require medical attention.

Blisters

Blisters are thin "bubbles" which form on skin damaged by friction or heat. They are caused by tissue fluid (serum) leaking into the burnt area just under the surface of the skin.

During healing, new skin forms at the base of the blister underneath the serum, the serum is reabsorbed and, eventually, the outer layer of skin peels off. Never break a blister; you will increase the risk of infection.

Unless a blister breaks or is likely to be further damaged, it requires no treatment. If it does need protection, apply a dressing large enough to extend well beyond the edges of the burnt area.

Clothing on Fire

Clothing may be set on fire by standing too close to an electric, gas or open fire or by carelessness in the kitchen. Without prompt help the result is widespread severe burning, shock and possible death. If the accident occurs indoors prevent a conscious casualty from panicking and rushing outside; the movement and/or breeze outside will fan the flames.

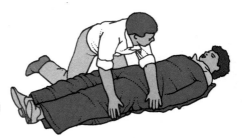

You should lay the casualty down as soon as possible to prevent flames sweeping upwards and quickly put out the flames by dousing the casualty with water or other *non-flammable* liquid. Alternatively, wrap the casualty tightly in

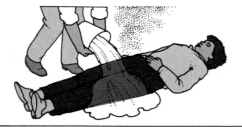

a coat, curtain, blanket (not the cellular type), rug or other heavy fabric then lay the person flat on the ground. This starves the flames of oxygen and puts them out.

Do not use nylon or other inflammable materials to smother the flames.

Do not roll the casualty along the ground as this can cause burning of previously unharmed areas.

If your own clothes have caught fire and help is not immediately available, extinguish the flames by wrapping yourself up tightly in suitable material (see above) and lying down.

Dry Burns and Scalds

These are the most common types of burns both in the home and in industry and they are a major cause of accidental death, particularly amongst children and the elderly.

Burns and scalds must be cooled as soon as possible in order to prevent further damage to underlying tissues and to alleviate pain, swelling and the possibility of shock. The most effective method of cooling is to flood the area gently with cold water.

Any clothing which has been soaked in boiling fluid should be removed as soon as it begins to cool. Cooled, dry, burnt clothing should not be removed because doing so may introduce an infection.

Very small burns or scalds can generally be treated on site. However, if you are in any doubt about the severity of the injury, or if the casualty is an infant or a sick or elderly person, always seek medical advice.

NB Friction burns should be treated as minor burns unless the skin is broken. If the skin is broken see *Minor External Bleeding*, p. 67.

General Symptoms and Signs
● Severe pain in and around the injured area if the burn is superficial. The area may be numb if the burn is deep.
● Redness, swelling of area, and sometimes blistering.
● Grey, charred, peeling skin around a severe burn.
● Symptoms and signs of shock (see p. 90). The degree of shock will relate directly to the extent of the injury.

Aim

Reduce the effect of the heat, prevent infection, relieve pain and minimise shock. Arrange urgent removal to hospital if burns are severe or extensive.

General Treatment
FOR MINOR BURNS AND SCALDS

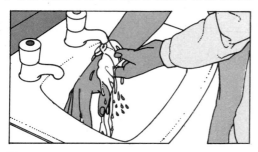

1 Reassure the casualty. Place the injured part under slowly running cold water or immerse it in cold water for 10 minutes — longer if the pain persists.

If no water is available, any cold, harmless liquid such as milk or beer can be used instead.

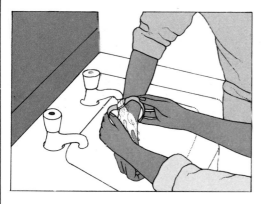

2 Gently remove any rings, watches, belts, shoes or other constricting clothing from the injured area *before* it starts to swell.

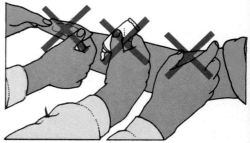

3 Dress the area with clean, preferably sterile, non-fluffy material (see *Dressings* pp. 172 – 5).

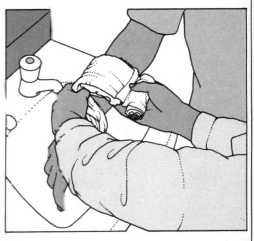

Do Not use adhesive dressings.

Do Not apply lotions, ointments or fat to injury.

Do Not break blisters, remove any loose skin or otherwise interfere with the injured area.

4 If in doubt about the severity of the injury seek medical aid.

General Treatment
FOR SEVERE BURNS AND SCALDS

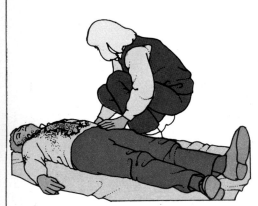

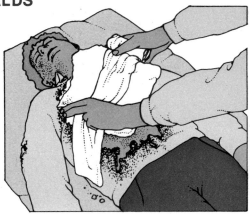

1 Lay the casualty down and make comfortable. Protect the burnt area from contact with the ground, if you can.

2 Gently remove any rings, watches, belts or constricting clothing from the injured area *before* it starts to swell.

3 Carefully remove any clothing soaked in boiling fluid after it has begun to cool.

Do Not remove anything that is sticking to a burn.

4 Cover the injured area with a sterile, unmedicated dressing or similar non-fluffy material and secure with a bandage (see *Dressings* pp. 172 – 5).

Do Not apply lotions, ointments or fat to injury.

Do Not break blisters, remove any loose skin or otherwise interfere with the injured area.

Burns in the Mouth and Throat

Burns to the mouth and throat usually result from drinking very hot liquid, swallowing corrosive chemicals or inhaling very hot air. These injuries are very serious because the tissues in the throat swell quickly and can close the airway making it difficult, if not impossible, for the casualty to breathe. As a result there is a real danger of asphyxia (see p. 45). In this situation it is particularly important to prevent the casualty panicking thereby worsening the situation.

Symptoms and Signs
● Casualty complains of severe pain in the injured area.
● Damaged skin around the mouth.
● Difficulty in breathing.
● Possible unconsciousness.
● Symptoms and signs of shock (see p. 90).

Aim
Arrange removal to hospital.

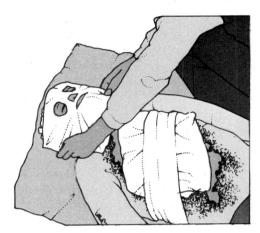
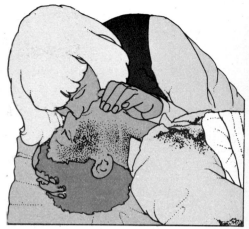

5 For facial burns, make a mask from a clean, dry, preferably sterile, piece of material (a pillow case is useful). Cut holes for the nose, mouth and eyes.

6 Immobilise a badly burned limb (see Fractures, pp. 106 – 127).

7 To minimise shock, treat as on p. 90.

If the casualty is conscious, give sips of cold water at frequent intervals to replace lost fluid.

8 If breathing and heartbeat stop, begin resuscitation immediately (see pp. 18 – 21).

9 If the casualty is unconscious but breathing normally, place in the Recovery Position (see p. 24).

10 Remove to hospital immediately maintaining the treatment position; transport as a stretcher case if necessary.

Treatment

1 Reassure the casualty.

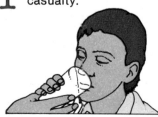

2 If the casualty is conscious, give sips of cold water at frequent intervals.

3 Remove any constricting clothing or jewellery from around the neck and chest.

4 If breathing and heartbeat stop, begin resuscitation immediately (see pp. 18 – 21).

5 If the casualty is unconscious but breathing normally, place in the Recovery Position (see p. 24).

6 To minimise shock, treat as on p. 90.

7 Remove to hospital immediately maintaining the treatment position; transport as a stretcher case if necessary.

Chemical Burns

Certain substances are irritating to the skin and contact with them can cause severe damage to the tissues; eyes are particularly vulnerable. Apart from the local effects, a few chemicals may be absorbed through the skin and cause widespread and sometimes fatal damage within the body.

Strong corrosives and chemicals will be found in industry but some household goods such as caustic soda, bleaches, household cleaners and paint strippers can cause chemical burns.

While prompt action with this type of burn is important, you should *always* consider your own safety before approaching the casualty.

Symptoms and Signs
● Casualty may complain that skin is stinging.
● Skin may appear stained or reddened and blistering and peeling may develop.

Aim
Identify and remove the harmful chemical as quickly as possible. Do not waste time looking for the antidote unless it is immediately available. Arrange urgent removal to hospital.

Treatment

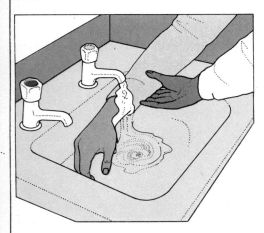

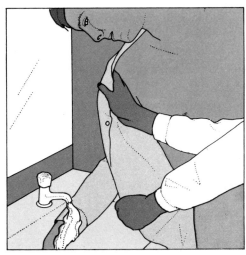

1 Flood the affected area with slowly running cold water for at least 10 minutes to prevent further damage to the burned tissue.

NB Make sure the water drains away freely and safely as it will be contaminated by the chemical which caused the burn.

2 Gently remove any contaminated clothing while flooding the injured area; make sure you do not contaminate yourself.

3 Continue treatment for severe burns, p. 138.

4 Remove to hospital immediately; transport as a stretcher case if necessary.

Chemical Burns in the Eye

Corrosive chemicals, both liquid and solid, can easily enter the eye and rapidly damage its surface causing severe scarring and even blindness.

Aim
Wash away the chemicals as quickly as possible and remove to hospital. *Do not* allow the casualty to rub the eye.

Symptoms and Signs
- Intense pain in the affected eye.
- Damaged eye cannot tolerate light.
- Affected eye may be tightly closed.
- The eye may be reddened, swollen or watering excessively.

Treatment

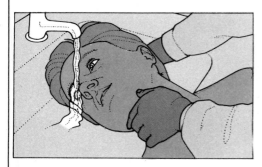

1 Hold the affected side of the casualty's face under gently running cold water so that the water drains away from the face. Alternatively, let the casualty put the affected side of the face in a bowl of cold water and ask the casualty to blink.

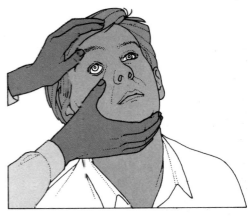

NB Check that both surfaces of the eyelids have been well-irrigated. If the eye is shut in a spasm of pain, you may have to pull the lids firmly, but gently, open.

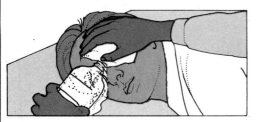

If this is not possible, sit or lay the casualty down with the head tilted back and turned towards the affected side. Protect the uninjured eye, gently open the eyelid of the affected eye and pour sterile water from an eye irrigator or a glass of tap water over it.

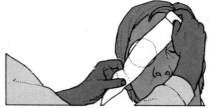

2 Lightly dress the eye with a sterile eye pad or, if this is not available, a pad of clean, non-fluffy material.

3 Remove to hospital immediately.

Electrical Burns

A burn may occur when electricity of a sufficiently high current and voltage passes through the body. Much of the damage occurs at, or close to, the points of entry and exit but, while only small burns may be visible, damage to the underlying tissues may be considerable. Electric shocks can also affect both breathing and heart action (see *Asphyxia* p. 58).

The most dangerous causes of electrical burns are high-voltage industrial machinery and lightning. Electricity in high-voltage industrial cables can jump or "arc" up to 18 m (20 yd) and kill you. So, do not approach the casualty unless you are officially informed that the current has been switched off (see p. 59).

Symptoms and Signs
● Redness, swelling, scorching or charring of the skin at both the entry and the exit points.
● Possible unconsciousness.
● Breathing and heartbeat may have stopped.
● Symptoms and signs of shock (see p. 90).

Aim
Separate the casualty from the source of injury, treat burns and arrange removal to hospital.

Treatment
1 Place a sterile dressing or pad of clean non-fluffy material over the burn. Secure with a bandage (see *Dressings* pp. 172 – 5).

Do Not apply lotions, ointments or fat to injury.

Do Not break blisters, remove any loose skin or otherwise interfere with the injured area.

2 To minimise shock, treat as on p. 90.

3 If breathing and heartbeat stop, begin resuscitation immediately (see pp. 18 – 21).

4 If the casualty becomes unconscious but is breathing normally, place in the Recovery Position (see p. 24).

5 Remove to hospital immediately maintaining the treatment position; transport as a stretcher case if necessary.

Sunburn

Direct exposure to the sun's rays may produce redness, itching and tenderness of the skin. It can vary from superficial burning to a more severe reaction in which the skin becomes lobster-red, blistered and painful.

Over-exposure to the sun's rays when it is very windy or the body is wet with sea-water or sweat can result in serious burns. However, sunburn can also occur even on a dull, overcast day in summer and in winter on high mountains when skiing because of the ultraviolet light.

Symptoms and Signs
● Casualty's skin will be red, tender and swollen with possible blistering.
● Affected skin will feel hot.

Aim
Remove casualty to a cool place and seek medical aid if burns are severe.

Treatment
1 Remove the casualty to the shade and cool the skin by sponging gently with cold water.

2 Give the casualty sips of cold water at frequent intervals.

3 For extensive blistering, seek medical aid immediately.

Do Not break blisters.

Snow Blindness and Welder's Flash

When the eyes are exposed to glare produced by the reflection of the sun on snow or concrete for too long, the cornea of the eye can be injured. This is a very painful condition and can take as long as a week to subside. It can easily be prevented by wearing dark glasses.

This condition can also result from the ultraviolet light produced by welding. Most protective helmets and goggles worn by welders give complete protec-

tion but careless use may expose a worker's eyes to a flash from an adjacent torch.

Symptoms and Signs

These normally appear some time after exposure to glare or welding flash.
- Casualty complains of intense pain in the affected eyes; eyes may feel as if they are full of sand or pepper.
- Affected eyes will be red, watering and sensitive to light.

Treatment

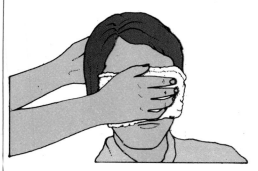

1 Bathe the eyes with cold water (see p. 141).

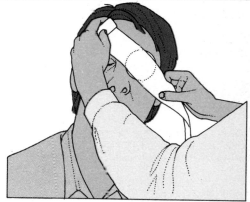

2 Lightly dress both eyes with eye pads or similar pads of clean, non-fluffy material.

3 If in doubt about the severity of the injury, seek medical aid immediately.

EFFECTS OF EXTREMES OF TEMPERATURE

Both extremes of temperature, excessive heat and cold, can damage the skin and other tissues of the body. In severe exposure, death may result.

Our bodies operate most efficiently within a narrow temperature range 36 – 37°C (97 – 99°F) with an average of 37°C (98.6°F). In order to keep a constant temperature, the body must retain its heat when the surrounding temperature is cool, and lose heat when the environment becomes hot.

The capillaries and sweat glands present in the skin are involved in temperature regulation. Part of the brain acts as a thermostat to achieve the balance between the heat gained by the body and the heat lost to the surroundings. In addition to this, the water vapour breathed out from the lungs helps to cool the body. However, this temperature regulation may be inadequate particularly in the very young or the elderly.

Temperature is affected by and can in part be regulated by:
* Insulation in the form of clothing or an artificially controlled environment (e.g., central heating or air conditioning).
* Food intake in the form of high-energy foods which produce heat or fluids which replace fluid lost through evaporation of sweat.
* Physical activity which produces heat. Over-exertion in hot climates can lead to heat exhaustion.

Methods of Producing Heat

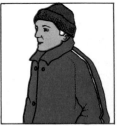
Warm clothing

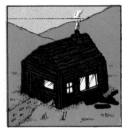
Heated shelter

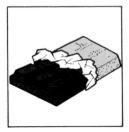
High-energy foods

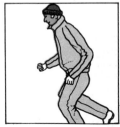
Physical activity

The Effects of Cooling

The body temperature falls when the environmental temperature is very low or during immersion in cold water. When this happens the following reactions take place:
* The skin capillaries contract making the person look pale and at the same time reducing the blood flow to the skin so that less heat is lost from the body surface.
* Shivering occurs — the skeletal muscles contract and relax rapidly (without us willing them to do so) and more heat is generated in the muscles.

Two conditions can arise from cooling: *hypothermia* where the whole body is affected by general cooling and *frostbite* where parts of the body, particularly the extremities, are affected locally.

Hypothermia

This is a condition which develops when the body temperature falls below about 35°C (95°F). Moderate hypothermia can normally be reversed and recovery will be complete. However, recovery is unlikely if the body temperature falls below 26 – 24°C (75 – 70°F).

NB A special thermometer is required to read such low temperatures.

Hypothermia occurs when the environmental temperature is very low but it can develop when temperatures are above freezing. It is commonly caused by: prolonged immersion in cold water; inadequate protection against a cold environment, particularly if the casualty is exhausted, wearing wet clothes or at a high altitude; or simply from general exposure to cold by being in an unheated or poorly heated house for a long period.

The ability of the body to protect itself from the cold is lessened by alcohol or drugs. Certain medical conditions such as diabetes may also be a contributory factor.

The onset of the effects of cold may pass unnoticed and their severity may vary with the age and physical condition of the individual, both of which govern the ability to resist chilling.

The Effects of Hypothermia

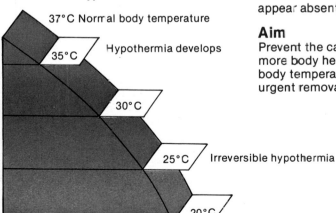

37°C Normal body temperature

35°C Hypothermia develops

30°C

25°C Irreversible hypothermia

20°C

Symptoms and Signs

General cooling causes the inner body temperature to drop and the casualty passes through several stages of discomfort and disability. Death may occur in a few hours or more rapidly in the case of immersion.

The different stages of hypothermia are as follows:
● Casualty complains of feeling miserably cold.
● Casualty's skin becomes pale, although infants may be pink and appear deceptively healthy (see over).
● Casualty feels abnormally cold to the touch.
● Intense and uncontrollable shivering (rigor) may appear.
● Shivering decreases and may be replaced by lack of muscle co-ordination and slurred speech.
● General comprehension of the situation is dulled and the casualty may become irrational.
● Pulse and respiration rate slow down.
● Loss of consciousness: breathing and heartbeat become increasingly difficult to detect.

NB *Never* assume that a casualty suffering from hypothermia is dead even if breathing and heartbeat appear absent.

Aim

Prevent the casualty from losing any more body heat and help to regain normal body temperature gradually. Arrange urgent removal to hospital.

Treatment

1 Place insulating material around the casualty covering the body, head and neck but *not* the face; lay the casualty down.

If the casualty is unconscious, place in the Recovery Position (see p. 24).

Do Not place the casualty's hands or arms in direct contact with the body as this draws heat off the body.

2 Remove casualty from the cold environment or high altitude. Place in a shelter or move to a warm room.

3 If the casualty's clothing is wet and adequate dry clothing is available, remove wet garments and replace them. If no dry clothing is available, leave wet clothes on and cover the casualty with waterproof material and additional insulation if available.

4 Give the conscious casualty hot sweet drinks.

5 If breathing and heartbeat stop or have stopped, begin resuscitation (see pp. 18 – 21).

NB A casualty with severe hypothermia may have a very slow heartbeat which is difficult to detect and an imperceptible breathing rate. Therefore, *always check for heartbeat for at least one minute before commencing External Chest Compression*. In severe hypothermia, premature External Chest Compression is particularly dangerous.

6 Examine the casualty for frostbite and treat as necessary.

7 Remove to hospital.

Do Not give the casualty any alcohol.

Do Not rub or massage the limbs or encourage the casualty to take any exercise.

If medical help is not readily available, apply gentle heat to the patient to prevent a further drop in temperature. Place hot water bottles wrapped in a towel or clothing on to the casualty's trunk but *not* the extremities.

HYPOTHERMIA IN INFANTS

Babies can suffer from hypothermia as they have difficulty in regulating their body temperatures. A baby with hypothermia may look very healthy so that its behaviour may be the only indication. Follow the treatment described above.

Symptoms and Signs

● The baby is unusually quiet, drowsy and limp.
● The baby will refuse food.
● Usually, the face, hands and feet are bright pink and healthy-looking.

HYPOTHERMIA IN THE ELDERLY

In addition to being less able to regulate their body temperatures, the elderly and infirm are often unable to look after themselves — they go without adequate food and heat and may not feel like moving about. In the aged, hypothermia may be mistaken for a stroke or heart attack. Treat as described above.

Frostbite

Frostbite occurs when the extremities of the body, most frequently the ears, nose, chin, hands and feet, are exposed to prolonged or intense cold. It may be *superficial*, freezing the skin only or *deep*, freezing both the skin and the underlying tissues. In severe cases gangrene of the affected parts may develop.

In the early stages it is not possible to differentiate between the two types. The initial symptoms and signs listed below are common to both. Frostbite may be accompanied by hypothermia; this should be treated before frostbite.

Symptoms and Signs
● Casualty complains of prickling pain in affected part, followed by gradual numbness.
● Movement of the affected part may be impaired.
● The skin feels hard and stiff.
● The skin appears wax-white or a mottled-blue colour.

Aim
Warm the affected area *slowly* and naturally to prevent further tissue destruction. Arrange removal to hospital.

Treatment

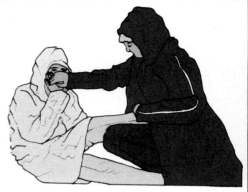

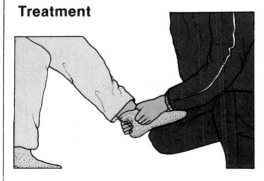

1 Remove to shelter and gently remove any clothing or covering from the affected area.

2 Remove anything of a constrictive nature, such as rings or watches.

3 Immediately re-warm the affected parts by skin-to-skin heat transfer from a warm part of the casualty or yourself. The hands may be placed in the casualty's armpits and the feet may be placed in your armpits. Cover frostbitten ears, nose or face with warm hands until colour and sensation return.

4 Place the injured part in hot water (tolerable to your elbow), if available.

Do Not let the casualty walk on a "defrosted" foot.

5 If re-warming reverses the signs within an hour stop the treatment but do not let the casualty be re-exposed to cold because the circulation has been damaged.

6 Elevate the affected parts to relieve swelling and pain.

7 Lightly cover the affected parts with soft dressings.

8 Remove to hospital.

Do Not rub or massage the affected parts.

Do Not break blisters or apply ointments or medications to the injured area.

Do Not re-warm by dry or radiant heat.

The Effects of Overheating

During strenuous exercise heat is released in the muscles and distributed to all parts of the body by the blood causing the general body temperature to rise. When this happens, the body reacts immediately to lose heat.

● The skin capillaries enlarge (dilate), so that more blood is carried to the surface allowing heat to be lost. This diversion of blood to the skin makes the person look hot and flushed.

● The sweat glands produce more sweat which evaporates and cools the body.

● Breathing increases and more heat is lost from the lungs.

Two conditions can arise from over-heating, heat exhaustion and heatstroke. *Heat exhaustion* usually affects people performing physical exercise in hot, moist climates especially if they do not replace the fluid and salt lost in sweat.

Heatstroke and rapid unconsciousness can occur during exposure to extreme heat or high humidity with no air current. The body temperature may rise as high as 40°C (104°F) because of a person's inability to sweat.

Heat Exhaustion

This is a condition caused by loss of salt and water from the body. It is more common in persons unaccustomed to working in a very hot, humid environment although in elderly persons, it may follow a debilitating illness. The condition can be aggravated by a stomach upset with diarrhoea and vomiting.

Symptoms and Signs

● Casualty may feel exhausted but restless.

● Casualty may have a headache and feel tired, dizzy and nauseated.

● Muscular cramps in the lower limbs and abdomen, caused by salt deficiency.

● Casualty's face will be pale and the skin will feel cold and clammy.

● Breathing becomes fast and shallow.

● Pulse is rapid and weak.

● Temperature remains normal or falls.

● Casualty may faint on any sudden movement.

Aim

Remove the casualty to a cooler environment and replace lost fluids and minerals. Seek medical aid.

Treatment

1 Lay the casualty down in a cool place.

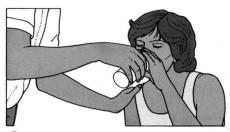

2 If the casualty is conscious, give sips of cold water to drink.

If the casualty is sweating profusely, has cramps, diarrhoea and/or is vomiting, add half a teaspoonful of salt to each ½ litre (1 pint) of water.

3 If the casualty becomes unconscious, but is breathing normally, place in the Recovery Position (see p. 24).

4 Seek medical aid.

Heatstroke

Heatstroke is caused by a very high environmental temperature or a feverish illness such as malaria, that leads to a greatly raised body temperature. It develops when the body can no longer control its temperature by sweating and can occur quite suddenly. It can develop in people of any age who have been exposed to heat and high humidity for too long and who are unaccustomed to them; or from prolonged confinement in a hot atmosphere. Anyone suffering from heatstroke should always receive medical attention.

Symptoms and Signs
● Casualty complains of headache, dizziness and of feeling hot.
● Casualty becomes restless.
● Unconsciousness may develop rapidly and become very deep.
● Casualty will be hot with a temperature of 40°C (104°F) or more and will look flushed although skin remains dry.
● Pulse is full and bounding; the breathing may be noisy.

Aim
Reduce the casualty's temperature as quickly as possible and seek medical aid.

Treatment
1 Move the casualty to a cool environment and remove the casualty's clothing.

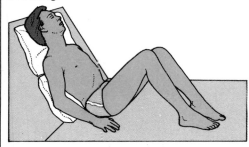

2 If the casualty is conscious, place in a half-sitting position with the head and shoulders supported.

If the casualty is unconscious but breathing normally, place in the Recovery Position (see p. 24).

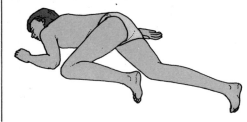

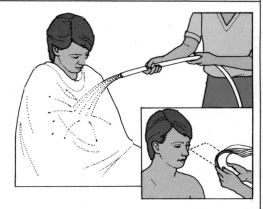

3 Wrap the casualty in a cold, wet sheet and keep it wet. Direct currents of air on to the casualty by fanning with a magazine, book or an electric fan until the casualty's temperature drops to 38°C (101°F).

4 Seek medical aid immediately.

If the casualty's temperature reduces, cover the casualty with a dry sheet and remove to an air-conditioned room if possible.

If the casualty's temperature rises again, repeat steps 3 and 4 above.

POISONING

A poison is any substance that, if taken into the body in sufficient quantity, can cause temporary or permanent damage. Instances of alleged poisoning occur in the United Kingdom each year involving both children and adults and some of them are fatal. Whilst some cases are attempted suicides, others are accidental and involve substances in everyday use. Whatever the cause of poisoning, medical aid should always be sought as soon as possible. *Never* attempt to make the casualty vomit; it is ineffective and you may worsen the situation.

THE DIGESTIVE SYSTEM

Food is broken down in the mouth, stomach and intestines by digestive juices secreted by various glands. It is taken in at the mouth and travels down the gullet (oesophagus) until it reaches the stomach. After partial digestion in the stomach, food then passes into the small intestine in small amounts. Here it is broken down into simple substances which are absorbed by the blood. The residue, consisting largely of vegetable fibres, enters the large intestine where accompanying water and mineral salts are absorbed. The final waste products are then eliminated from the body through the rectum at the anus.

The liver acts as a chemical factory which, amongst other functions, inactivates some poisons. The kidneys rid the blood of many impurities.

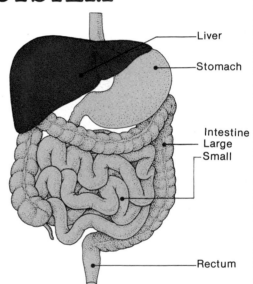

Liver

Stomach

Intestine
Large
Small

Rectum

How Poisons Enter the Body

Poisons can enter the body in a number of ways either accidentally or intentionally:
● Through the mouth by eating or drinking poisonous substances.
● Through the lungs by inhaling household or industrial gases (not North Sea gas; it is not poisonous), chemical vapours or fumes from fires, stoves and petrol-engine exhausts.

● By injection into the skin as the result of bites from some animals, insects, poisonous fish or reptiles or by hypodermic syringe.
● By absorption through the skin through contact with poisonous sprays such as pesticides and insecticides.

How Poisons Act

When in the body poisons act in various ways. Once in the bloodstream, some poisons work on the central nervous system preventing breathing, heart action and other vital life processes. Other poisons act by displacing the oxygen in the blood and preventing its distribution to the tissues.

Swallowed (ingested) poisons also react directly on the food passages resulting in vomiting, pain and often diarrhoea. Corrosive poisons may severely burn the lips, mouth, gullet and stomach thus causing intense pain.

General Symptoms and Signs

These vary depending on the nature of the poison and the method of entry into the body.

● Information from the casualty or an onlooker suggesting contact with a poison. Try to ascertain exactly what was involved and if swallowed, when and how much was taken.

● Presence of a container near the casualty known to hold or have held poison or a poisonous plant.
● Casualty may be delirious and have convulsions without previous history of such conditions.
● Symptoms and signs of asphyxia (see p. 45).
● Unconsciousness may develop.
● If the poison was swallowed, the casualty may begin retching or vomiting or suffer from diarrhoea.
● Burns around the casualty's mouth after contact with corrosive poisons.

NB A casualty attempting suicide may dispose of any evidence which would aid diagnosis.

Aim

Maintain an open airway and get the casualty to medical aid or hospital as soon as possible.

General Treatment

1 Quickly ask the conscious casualty what has happened; remember that the casualty may lose consciousness at any time.

Do Not attempt to induce vomiting.

If the lips or mouth show signs of burning, cool them by giving the casualty water or milk to drink.

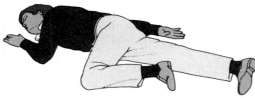

2 If the casualty is unconscious, but breathing normally, place in the Recovery Position (see p. 24).

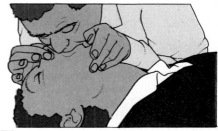

3 If breathing and heartbeat stop, begin resuscitation immediately (see pp. 18 – 21).

NB Take care not to contaminate yourself with any poison that may be around the casualty's mouth.

4 Remove to hospital immediately. Send any samples of vomit and containers such as bottles or pill boxes found nearby to the hospital with the casualty.

Household Poisons

Many substances found in and about the home can be poisonous. These include liquid soap, some cosmetics, fire-lighters, turpentine, bleach, glue, rat-poison, paint stripper, garden sprays and insecticides. Children are especially at risk from such materials since they may not or cannot be aware of the conse-quences of eating or drinking them.

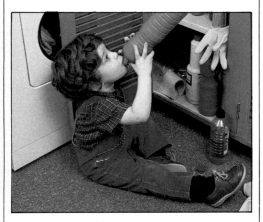

The symptoms and signs will vary according to the poison, although vomit-ing and abdominal pain are likely to occur in most cases. Treat the casualty as des-cribed on p. 151 and remove to hospital.

Children are also liable to take medi-cines and tablets found in medicine cabinets. While most household medi-cines and tablets are not dangerous if taken as directed, many are poisonous if the dosage is exceeded. Some of the more dangerous medicines include cap-sules and tablets which look like sweets, for example, certain iron tablets, junior aspirin (especially the coloured ones), tranquillisers and barbiturates.

NB Always make sure that all bottles and jars containing poisonous substances are clearly marked and kept out of reach of children.

Poisonous Plants

Certain plants, around our gardens as well as in the wild, are dangerous if eaten and some may cause allergic reactions if touched. Children, in particular, are attracted by the bright berries of many of these plants and eat them.

Laburnum (laburnum anagyroides), deadly nightshade (atropha belladonna) and death cap fungus (amanita phal-loides) are the more common examples of plants which can poison the system. The symptoms and signs of this type of poisoning are similar to those of food poisoning, see below. The severity of the condition will depend upon how much of the plant has been taken. If you suspect that a casualty has eaten a poisonous plant or berries it is important that you maintain an open airway and remove the casualty to hospital immediately.

There are very few plants in the United Kingdom which cause a reaction when touched. However, contact with those that are likely to cause a reaction may only result in a mild rash or swollen eyelids.

Food Poisoning

This is caused by food becoming con-taminated by bacteria and being stored or cooked incorrectly. The most common bacteria are: staphylococci, which multi-ply in the food and produce a poisonous substance (toxin); or salmonellae, which multiply in the bowel and cause a dysen-tery-like illness. Salmonella is infectious and can be passed through poor personal and kitchen hygiene.

Symptoms and Signs

Staphylococcal poisoning
These symptoms and signs will appear within two to six hours of eating the

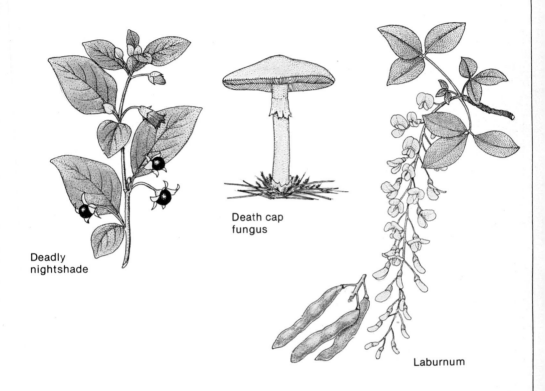

Deadly
nightshade

Death cap
fungus

Laburnum

contaminated food.
● Casualty will feel nauseated and may already be vomiting.
● Casualty may be suffering from abdominal pain and may have a headache.
● Diarrhoea may develop at a later stage.
● Symptoms and signs of shock (see p. 90)

Salmonella Poisoning

The symptoms and signs of Salmonella poisoning may appear within a few hours of eating the food or be delayed for a day or two.
● Casualty develops a fever.
● Casualty will be suffering from diarrhoea.
● Casualty may feel nauseated and begin vomiting.

● Casualty may be suffering from abdominal pain.
● Symptoms and signs of shock (see p. 90).

Aim

Seek medical aid.

Treatment

See general treatment of poisons.

1 Keep the casualty at rest.

2 Give the casualty plenty of fluids.

3 If in doubt about the casualty's condition, arrange removal to hospital.

Drug Poisoning

This condition is caused by accidental overdose or drug abuse. Drug abuse may be broadly defined as the self-administration of a drug in a manner that is not in accordance with approved medical or social patterns. Drugs can be inhaled, swallowed or injected into the body. A regular drug abuser may show signs of continuous use of hypodermic injections. These marks will usually be on the front of the forearm near the elbow, although other places are used. The veins in the area will become inflamed and infected.

Drugs commonly abused are: narcotics (e.g., heroin); depressants (e.g., barbiturates and tranquillisers); stimulants (e.g., amphetamines) and hallucinogens (eg., L.S.D.). In addition there is solvent inhalation (e.g., "glue-sniffing").

Symptoms and Signs
These will vary according to the drug and the quantity taken. Vomiting will not always appear immediately but you should watch for it. The pupils of the eyes may be abnormally dilated or contracted.

Narcotics
These are usually injected but can be taken in tablet form or inhaled.
- Breathing becomes difficult and eventually will cease.
- Casualty may have injection marks on the front of one or both arms.

Depressants
- Breathing will be shallow
- Casualty's skin will feel cold and clammy.
- Weak and rapid pulse.
- Possible unconsciousness.

Stimulants
- Casualty will be excitable and sweating profusely.
- Casualty may be suffering from tremors and hallucinations.

Hallucinogens
- Casualty will be anxious and sweating.
- Casualty may be behaving strangely.

Aspirin Overdose
- Casualty has abdominal pain, and may be vomiting. Vomit may be blood-stained.
- Casualty may be depressed and drowsy.
- Casualty may complain of "ringing" in the ears (tinnitus).
- Difficulty in breathing.
- Casualty will be sweating profusely.
- Full pulse.

Treatment
Follow the general treatment for poisoning. Arrange urgent removal to hospital and be prepared to resuscitate.

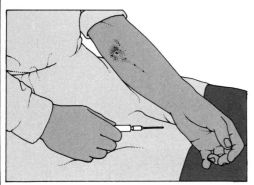

Injection marks and swollen veins on the forearms are common signs of drug abuse.

Alcohol Poisoning

Alcohol is a drug that depresses the central nervous system. It affects different people in different ways. One drink usually only produces a slight change in mood. As the intake continues, however, the drug affects the areas of higher reasoning within the brain — those that control restraint and judgement. As the concentration of alcohol in the blood increases, the behaviour of the drinker becomes exaggerated and co-ordination will be impaired. Eventually, the mental and physical abilities are deeply disturbed and unconsciousness will develop.

Symptoms and Signs
● Casualty's breath may smell of alcohol.
● Casualty may be vomiting.
● Casualty may be partly conscious or already unconscious. If unconscious you may be able to rouse the casualty, but the casualty will lapse into unconsciousness again quite quickly.

In early stages of unconsciousness:
● Casualty will be breathing deeply.
● Face will be moist and flushed.
● Pulse will be full and bounding.

In later stages of unconsciousness:
● Pulse may become rapid but weak.
● Breathing will be shallow.
● Casualty's face will feel dry and look bloated.
● Eyes will be bloodshot and pupils may be dilated.

Aim
Ensure an open airway; arrange removal to hospital if the casualty is unconscious.

Treatment

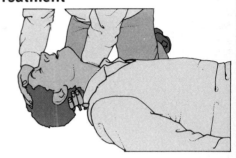

1 Maintain an open airway (see p. 15).

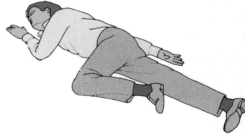

2 If casualty becomes unconscious or vomiting is likely, place in the Recovery Position (see p. 24)

3 If in doubt about the casualty's condition, remove to hospital.

Industrial Poisons

Some people may be in contact with dangerous chemicals or gases at their work places by, for example, the failure of a chemical plant or spillage of corrosive substances.

Amongst the most common industrial poisons are gases. These are usually classed as: irritants (e.g., ammonia and nitrous fumes); asphyxiants (e.g., carbon dioxide); toxic gases (e.g., carbon monoxide and hydrogen cyanide gas); and toxic vapours (e.g., those given off by volatile chemicals such as carbon-tetra-chloride or trichloroethylene).

There are so many different poisonous substances in use that it is impossible to give a comprehensive list. Any factory using potentially dangerous chemicals or gases must display notices indicating any special action to be taken in case of accidents (see *Accidents Involving Dangerous Chemicals* p. 170). Therefore, if you are called to an industrial accident involving dangerous substances, contact a responsible works official. Always obey any safety regulations to avoid further injury to yourself and the casualty.

Remember that any casualty suffering from the effects of gas or toxic fumes needs air. Take great care to prevent yourself being overcome by any fumes that remain in the area. Never attempt to rescue a casualty trapped in an enclosed space unless equipped with, and practised in the use of, breathing apparatus and life-lines.

Severe Allergic Reactions (Anaphylactic Shock)

Anaphylactic shock is a massive allergic reaction which can develop within a few seconds or minutes of an injection of a drug or insect sting to which the casualty is sensitive. More rarely it follows the ingestion of an allergen such as penicillin, in which case the reaction will be slower.

Symptoms and Signs
● Symptoms and signs of shock (see p. 90).
● Casualty will feel nauseated and may be vomiting.
● Casualty complains that chest feels tight.
● Difficulty in breathing — casualty may be wheezing and gasping for air.
● Casualty may be sneezing.
● There may be facial swelling especially around the eyes.
● Pulse will be rapid.
● Unconsciousness may develop.

Aim
Arrange urgent removal to hospital and be prepared to resuscitate.

Treatment
See treatment for shock, p. 90.

1 Maintain an open airway. If breathing becomes difficult, place casualty in the Recovery Position (see p. 24).

2 If breathing and heartbeat stop, begin resuscitation immediately (see pp. 18 – 21).

3 Remove to hospital immediately.

FOREIGN BODIES

A "foreign body" means any extraneous matter that enters the body either through a wound in the skin (penetrating) or via one of the natural openings of the body (inserted or swallowed).

A penetrating foreign body can be anything that enters the body from a tiny splinter of wood or glass to a large wooden stake or piece of metal. It may be loose and easily removed without causing further pain or injury or it can be embedded. The latter may, in addition, be acting as a plug preventing blood loss (see p. 66).

Large foreign bodies embedded in the skin may produce a deep wound but small splinters cause little more than minor lacerations.

The main problem with injuries involving penetrating foreign bodies is that foreign bodies are rarely clean so that there is a high risk of infection (see *Wounds and Bleeding*, p. 68). Whatever their size or nature foreign bodies should be removed as soon as possible. The small loose ones may be removed by you but embedded foreign bodies *must* be removed at a hospital.

Loose Foreign Bodies

Most particles of loose grit can be washed out or removed with a clean swab or tweezers, and dressed.

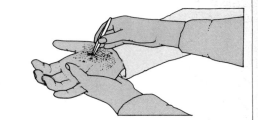

Embedded Foreign Bodies

If particles or objects are deeply embedded in the skin dress them, using a ring pad if necessary (see *Wounds and Bleeding* p. 66). Make the casualty as comfortable as possible and seek medical aid immediately. If the casualty becomes impaled on an immovable object such as a metal railing, the fire brigade, as well as an ambulance, will be required (see p. 35).

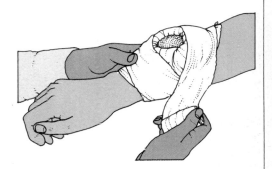

Swallowed Foreign Bodies

Smooth swallowed objects need not necessarily cause alarm. A sharp object on the other hand, can cause severe damage. In either case, always seek medical aid as soon as possible.

Splinters

Wood and metal splinters which have become embedded in the skin are probably the most common foreign bodies with which you will be confronted. They can generally be removed with tweezers as described below. However, if the splinter is deeply embedded, seek medical aid as soon as possible.

Symptoms and Signs
● Known contact with pieces of wood, metal or glass.
● Visible indication of embedded foreign body.
● Pain and tenderness in the area.

Aim
Gently remove the splinter.

Treatment

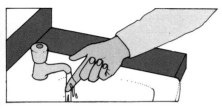

1 If the area around the splinter is dirty, cleanse it using soap and water (see *Wounds and Bleeding* p. 67).

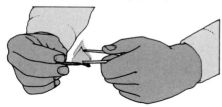

2 Sterilise a pair of tweezers by passing them through a flame.

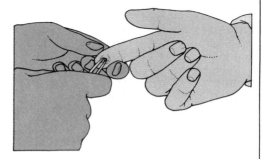

3 Gently try to pull the splinter out of the wound with tweezers. Hold the tweezers as near to the skin as possible and grasp the splinter; pull the splinter out in the opposite direction to that in which it entered the skin.

4 If the splinter does not come out easily or begins to break up, treat as an embedded foreign body (see p. 66) and seek medical aid.

Do Not probe the area to reach the splinter.

NB Make sure the casualty's tetanus inoculation is up-to-date (see p. 69) because splinters are rarely clean.

Foreign Bodies in the Nose

These are usually encountered in very young children who try to insert various objects such as pebbles or marbles into their noses. Smooth objects may just be lodged in the nose but a sharp object can easily damage the tissues of the nose. Do not attempt to remove the object but remove the casualty to hospital.

Symptoms and Signs
● Casualty has difficulty in breathing through the nose.
● Occasionally, nose appears swollen.
● Discharge (often blood-stained) appearing from one or both sides of the nose.

Aim
Reassure the casualty and remove to hospital as soon as possible.

Treatment
1 Keep the casualty quiet and advise to breathe through the mouth.

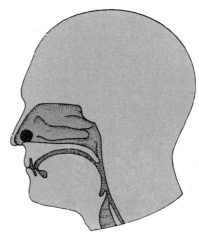

2 Remove to hospital.

Do Not attempt to remove the foreign body.

Foreign Bodies in the Ear

These are most common in young children. They can cause some temporary deafness but deep penetration can damage the eardrum. Alternatively, insects may become lodged in a person's ear.

Symptoms and Signs
● Casualty complains of pain in the ear.
● Casualty may feel vibrations if an insect is inside the ear.
● Hearing on affected side impaired.

Aim
Remove the casualty to hospital.

Treatment
1 Reassure the casualty.

2 If a foreign body is suspected, *do not* attempt to dislodge it as probing may perforate the eardrum.

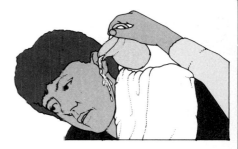

3 If it is an insect, gently flood the ear with tepid water to float it out.

4 Remove to hospital.

Foreign Bodies in the Eye

All eye injuries are potentially serious because particles may perforate the eyeball resulting in internal damage and possible infection.

Particles of dust or grit or loose eyelashes are the most common foreign bodies found in the eyes. They stick to the outer surface of the eyeball or become lodged under the eyelid, normally the upper lid, causing considerable discomfort and inflammation. In most cases these can easily be removed. However, *do not* attempt to remove a foreign body if it is on the coloured part of the eye (pupil and iris) or embedded in the eyeball. In these cases, seek medical aid immediately.

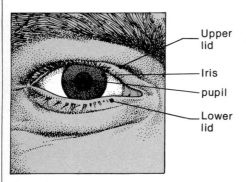

Upper lid

Iris

pupil

Lower lid

Symptoms and Signs
- Casualty's eye is painful and itches.
- Casualty's vision may be impaired.
- Watering of affected eye.
- Casualty's eye is red.

Aim
Remove particle gently. If unsuccessful, remove casualty to hospital.

Treatment
1 Advise the casualty *not* to rub the eye (the casualty will almost certainly be doing so).

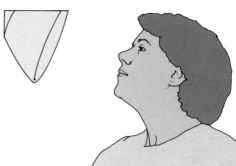

2 Ask the casualty to sit down in a chair facing the light and lean back.

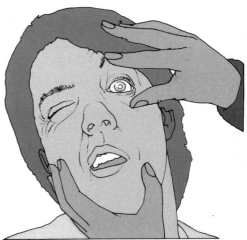

3 Stand behind the casualty. Hold the chin in one hand and use the index finger and thumb of your other hand to separate the affected lids. Ask the casualty to look right, left, up and down so that you can examine every part of the eye properly.

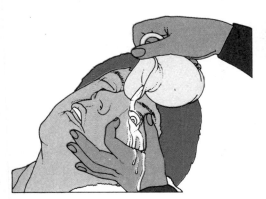

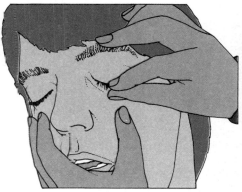

4 If you can see the foreign body try to wash it out with a *sterile water solution* and an eye irrigator. If these are not available, irrigate the eye with tap water. Incline the head towards the injured side so that the water will drain out over the cheek away from the sound eye; pour water from a jug or place the casualty's head under a tap (see p. 141).

6 If the foreign body is under the upper lid, ask the casualty to look down. Grasp the eyelashes and pull the upper lid downwards and outwards over *the lower lid*. If the lashes of the lower lid do not brush the foreign body off, get the casualty to blink the eye under water in the hope that it will float off.

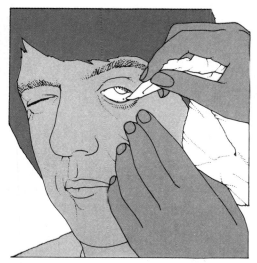

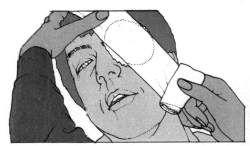

7 If you cannot remove the foreign body, cover the affected eye with an eye pad or a piece of gauze wrapped around a soft pad of cotton wool. Secure it lightly in position and seek medical aid.

If the foreign body is on the coloured part of the eye or it is embedded in or sticking to the eyeball *do not attempt to remove it*. Advise the casualty, not to move the eye. Cover it with an eye pad. If necessary prevent eye movement by covering both eyes. Remove to hospital. For treatment of chemicals in the eye see p. 141.

5 If this is unsuccessful or no water is available and the foreign body is *not* sticking to the eye, lift the foreign body off using a moistened swab or the damp corner of a clean handkerchief.

Insect Stings

Insects, such as bees, wasps and hornets or jellyfish such as Portuguese-Men-o-War cause stings which are more painful and alarming than they are dangerous. Some people, however, are allergic to the poison. Moreover, multiple stings from a swarm of insects can have a dangerous cumulative effect (see *Severe Allergic Reaction* p. 157). Stings in the mouth and throat may cause swelling leading to Asphyxia (see p. 45).

Symptoms and Signs
● Unexpected sharp pain; an insect may still be present.
● There will be swelling around the affected area with a central reddened puncture point.
● Possibility of shock depending on the degree of reaction (see p. 90).

Aim
Remove sting if present and attempt to reduce swelling and relieve pain. If the sting is inside the mouth remove the casualty to hospital immediately.

Treatment
FOR STINGS IN THE SKIN

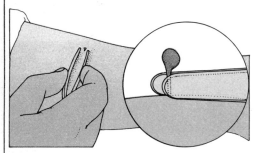

1 If the sting has been left embedded in the skin, hold tweezers as near to the skin as possible, grasp the sting and remove it (see p. 158).

Do Not squeeze the poison sac because this will force the remaining poison into the skin.

2 To relieve pain and swelling, apply a cold compress (see p. 176), surgical spirit or a solution of bicarbonate of soda. For jellyfish stings smooth calamine lotion into the affected area.

3 If pain and swelling persist or increase over the next day or so, advise the casualty to seek medical aid.

FOR INSECT STINGS INSIDE THE MOUTH OR THROAT

1 To reduce the swelling, give the casualty ice to suck. Alternatively, rinse the mouth with cold water or a solution of water and bicarbonate of soda, if available (1 teaspoon to each tumbler).

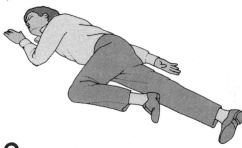

2 If breathing becomes difficult, place casualty in the Recovery Position (see p. 24).

3 Remove to hospital.

Fish Hooks in the Skin

Sometimes only the point of the hook enters the skin, in which case the hook can easily be removed. If, however, the barb is caught as well, do not try to remove it but seek medical aid. Only attempt to remove it if medical aid is not immediately available.

Aim

Gently remove the point and treat as a minor wound. Seek medical aid if the barb has penetrated.

Treatment

1 Cut the line from the fish hook.

2 If the barb is not caught in the skin, remove the hook and treat as a minor wound (see p. 67).

3 If the barb is caught in the skin, treat as an embedded foreign body (see p. 66) and seek medical aid.

IF MEDICAL AID IS NOT READILY AVAILABLE

1 Cut the line from the fish hook.

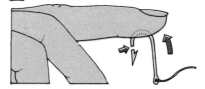

2 As long as there is no danger of damaging internal organs, push the hook through the skin until the barb protrudes, then cut through the shaft between the barb and the skin.

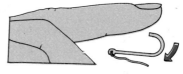

3 Gently withdraw the hook, clean the wound and cover with a dressing.

4 Seek medical aid to deal with any infection in the wound.

Swallowed Foreign Bodies

Children in particular often swallow small objects such as pins, coins or buttons. Most small smooth objects are unlikely to damage the intestine or cause choking. However, sharp objects such as pins or needles can damage the intestine. In either case you should seek medical aid or remove the casualty to hospital.

Symptoms and Signs
● History indicating that object has been swallowed.

Aim

Reassure the casualty and remove to hospital

Treatment

1 Reassure the casualty and the parents if the casualty is a child.

2 Remove to hospital.

Do Not give the casualty anything by mouth.

ACHES

An ache is a continuous dull pain. Some aches are symptomatic of another condition or injury and may be referred from some other part of the body.

While it is not always possible for you to diagnose the cause of the symptoms, you should attempt to provide temporary relief from the pain. However, the administration of medicines is beyond the scope of First Aid. On the other hand, if someone suffering from a minor ache is carrying some pain-killing tablets (*not* aspirin), the person may be able to deal with the ache in this way.

The aim of all treatment is to relieve discomfort. Treatments for the more common aches are described on the following pages; other conditions such as chest pain caused by heart attacks, are dealt with elsewhere in the book. It is important that you look out for any symptoms or signs mentioned and that you seek medical aid immediately if you notice them.

NB For treatment of minor illness see the companion book *Caring for the Sick*.

Headache

Common causes of headache are: sinusitis, the common cold, stress, eye strain, pressure and lack of sleep or food. However, injuries to the head or spine can also result in headaches.

Symptoms and Signs
● Pain anywhere in the head which may be constant, throbbing or intermittent.

Treatment
1 Place a cold compress (see p. 176) or covered hot-water bottle on the casualty's forehead whichever is preferred.

NB The casualty may take one or two own pain-killing tablets if available.

2 If practical, advise the casualty to lie down in a darkened room.

3 If the headache persists, or if it is accompanied by a feeling of nausea, vomiting, fever, stiff neck, disturbed vision, obvious head injury, confusion or gradual loss of consciousness, seek medical aid.

Migraine

These severe and at times incapacitating headaches sometimes come on for no apparent reason and cannot normally be traced to any particular disorder. However, they may follow lack of food, noise, heat, travelling, or emotional disturbances.

Migraine attacks are more severe than normal headaches but they are not as common and only the casualty will know if it is a migraine attack.

Symptoms and Signs
● Casualty may experience "flickering" vision — this can precede the headache.
● Casualty will be feeling nauseated and may already be vomiting.
● Intense throbbing headache which may only affect one side of the head.
● Casualty cannot tolerate light or noise.
● Casualty may look very pale.

Treatment
As for Headache, above.

Toothache

The most frequent cause of toothache is decay which has penetrated the enamel of a tooth. However, it can also be the result of an abscess, abnormal pressure from an incorrect bite or pain referred from somewhere else, for example, pain caused by inflammation of a facial nerve (neuralgia).

Symptoms and Signs
● Pain in the teeth or jaws, which may be constant, throbbing or intermittent. The pain may be made worse by cold or hot food and drink.

Treatment

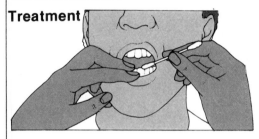

1 Dab the affected tooth with oil of cloves, if available, to deaden pain.

NB The casualty may take one or two own pain-killing tablets, if available.

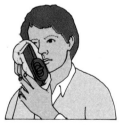

2 To relieve a severe or persistent toothache, hold a covered hot water bottle or heated pad against the affected side of the face.

3 If symptoms persist, or if there is fever or swelling around the tooth involved, advise the casualty to see the dentist or doctor without delay.

Earache

This can be very painful. It is often the result of an infection in or near the ear, for example, a boil in the ear canal or an abcessed tooth. The most common cause, however, particularly in children, is middle-ear infection caused by germs spreading from the throat to the middle ear. This type of infection may follow illnesses such as tonsillitis, measles or influenza. Earache can also occur when there is too much wax present in the ear canal or if there is a sudden change of pressure on the eardrum during air travel or underwater swimming.

Symptoms and Signs
● Constant or throbbing pain in the ear.

Treatment

1 To relieve a severe or persistent earache, hold a covered hot water bottle or heated pad against the affected ear.

NB The casualty may take one or two own pain-killing tablets, if available.

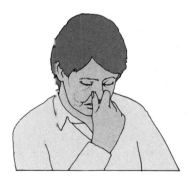

2 If earache is caused by a sudden change of pressure advise the casualty to hold the nose and close the mouth and then swallow or blow out the cheeks.

3 If the ache persists or if it is accompanied by discharge, fever, impaired hearing and/or balance, advise the casualty to seek medical aid immediately.

Neck Ache

Mild soreness or stiffness of the neck muscles may be caused by sitting or lying in one position for too long, exposure to draughts or nervous tension but it may also result from a viral illness or an injury such as "Whiplash" (see p. 114).

Symptoms and Signs
Pain anywhere in the neck increased by movement.

Treatment
1 To relieve pain, hold a covered hot water bottle or heated pad against the affected area and encourage gentle movement of the neck.

NB The casualty may take one or two own pain-killing tablets, if available.

2 If the symptoms persist or if they are accompanied by swelling, feelings of nausea and/or vomiting, headache, confusion and/or loss of consciousness or obvious injury, seek medical aid.

Back Ache

Pain in the back can be a symptom of various disorders. Some involve the back itself, for instance, a strain (see p. 129), poor posture or a displaced disc (see p. 132). In other cases, pain may be caused by disorders elsewhere in the body (e.g., kidney infection).

Symptoms and Signs
● Pain anywhere in the back.

Treatment
1 If caused by a strain treat as on p. 129. Otherwise place a covered hot water bottle on (see p. 176) the affected area.

NB The casualty may take one or two own pain-killing tablets, if available.

2 If the symptoms persist, there is a raised temperature, the urine has a strong smell or is bloodstained, there is trouble with the bowels and/or bladder, or a loss of movement or sensation in the legs, seek medical aid.

Abdominal Pain

There are many causes of abdominal pain including indigestion, colic, menstrual cramp, constipation and food poisoning. Generally, such pain is not considered serious if it lasts less than half an hour and there are no other symptoms such as headache, vomiting, fever or diarrhoea.

Symptoms and Signs
● Pain anywhere in the abdomen, which may be dull or sharp, constant or intermittent, localised or general.

Treatment
1 To relieve pain, place the casualty in a half-sitting position with the head and shoulders supported. Bend the knees and support in this position.

If menstrual cramps are suspected, the casualty may find walking about relieves the discomfort.

2 Place a covered hot-water bottle or a heated pad over the affected area.

3 If vomiting is likely place in the Recovery Position (see p. 24).

4 Keep the casualty lying down and comfortable. To minimise shock, treat as on p. 90.

5 If the pain lasts more than half an hour or you are in doubt about the casualty's condition, seek medical aid.

PROCEDURE AT MAJOR INCIDENTS

Major incidents are those in which a large number of casualties are involved. They can be natural, for example an earthquake, or involve human error, as in a road traffic accident. The number of casualties, and the sequence in which they will need to be treated, will vary according to the incident and the types of injury. Casualties may be trapped, thrown some distance or found wandering about in a dazed condition. In a major fire, injuries may be caused by people jumping out of a high building or being trapped in a smoke-filled room.

In any emergency, the way you approach the situation is important (see p. 33). This is especially true in a major incident and because a single First Aider cannot treat all the casualties at once, it is essential that a brief reconnaisance of the scene is made. You will need to find out: exactly what has happened; whether danger still threatens; how many casualties there are and what condition they are in. All this information must then be passed on to the emergency services immediately (see p. 35). If there is no further danger, you should then treat the casualties on site according to the priorities of breathing, bleeding and unconsciousness.

Remember, the general rule for dealing with any casualty in danger is: remove the danger from the casualty and, *only if this is not possible*, remove the casualty from the danger.

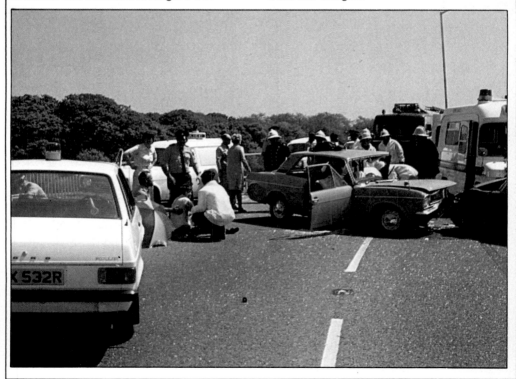

Road Traffic Accidents

The general principles for dealing with any major incident can best be illustrated by the procedure for dealing with casualties in a road traffic accident. The most important thing to remember is that you should not attempt to move a casualty unless absolutely necessary – leave it to the emergency services.

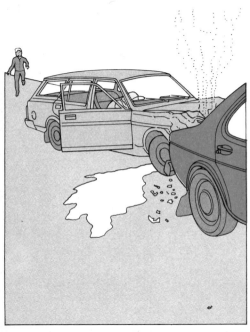

Taking calculated risks

In many road traffic accidents casualties may have to be moved in order to save lives. The decision to do so, however, should be *very* carefully considered, especially if the casualty is unconscious, because of the risk of spinal injury or severe internal bleeding.

Unless casualties are in danger of further injury, for instance from fire, or breathing and heartbeat have stopped, you should carry out a full examination to determine the extent of the injuries before moving them. Then, follow the procedure described opposite.

IMMEDIATE ACTION

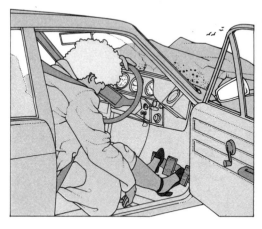

● Look for any indication of dangerous substances being present such as Hazchem warnings.
● Instruct someone to telephone the emergency services immediately (see *Calling for Assistance* p. 35).
● Do not pull casualties from the vehicle – this could result in further injuries.

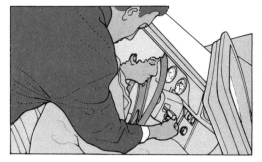

● Minimise the risk of fire by switching off the engine and, if you know how, disconnecting the battery because fires often begin in the wiring under the bonnet or dashboard. Do not allow anyone to smoke near the vehicle. If a diesel lorry, bus or car is involved, switch off the fuel supply – there is normally an emergency switch on the outside of the vehicle.

● Instruct bystanders to set up warning triangles at least 200 m (220 yd) from the accident; if no triangles are available, ask them to direct traffic.

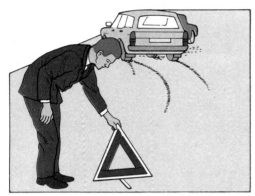

● Immobilise the car. If it is on four wheels apply the handbrake, put the car into gear and/or place blocks under the wheels. If the car is on its side and there are passengers inside, *do not try to right it*, just make sure that it will not roll over.

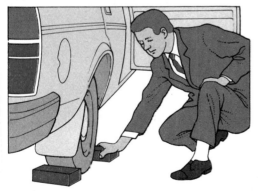

● Look inside the vehicle for any small children who may have fallen out of sight or be hidden under blankets or luggage. Check the area immediately surrounding the vehicle for any passengers who may have been thrown out of the vehicle or who may be wandering about . Ask a conscious casualty how many people were in the vehicle before the accident.

MOVING A CASUALTY

If the situation is such that a casualty needs to be moved then it must be done very carefully. The casualty should be immobilised as far as possible and you should make sure that you have enough people to support all parts of the body. If bystanders are helping you they must be given clear instructions on how the casualty is going to be moved. Each person should be aware of exactly what he or she is to do (see *Handling and Transport* pp. 192 – 209) and the removal should be carried out in one continuous movement if possible.

If a casualty is trapped under a vehicle and has to be removed before the emergency services arrive, because of the danger of fire for example, try to move the vehicle away from the casualty first. If this is not possible, immobilise the vehicle as described left, and move the casualty as gently as possible. Remember to note the exact position of the casualty or vehicle before moving either because the police may need this information later.

In all cases where you have decided against moving the casualty you should always be prepared to do so should the casualty's condition deteriorate or new danger threaten.

DEALING WITH TRAPPED CASUALTIES

Accident victims may be trapped in their vehicles by an impacted steering wheel, for instance. Such a casualty should be watched carefully because, if unconscious, the tongue may fall to the back of the throat and block the airway. To guard against this possibility, the casualty's head should be placed in the Open Airway Position (see p. 15). A trapped casualty must be observed continuously until the arrival of skilled help.

ACCIDENTS INVOLVING DANGEROUS SUBSTANCES

Accidents may be complicated by the spillage of dangerous liquids or the escape of toxic fumes, and any such incident should be approached with great care. Never make any rescue attempt unless you are sure that it is safe to do so; do not endanger yourself by coming into contact with a dangerous substance.

Most vehicles and containers carrying dangerous substances now display notices which signify exactly what is being carried. If you are in doubt about the meaning of the sign keep your distance, especially if there is any spillage. Make a careful note of the code and give the information to the emergency services. Keep bystanders well away from the scene and bear in mind the possibility that poisonous fumes may be given off. If this does occur, stand upwind of the accident so that any fumes are blown away from you.

Hazard Warnings

Vehicles carrying dangerous goods display hazard warning information panels indicating the substance being carried.

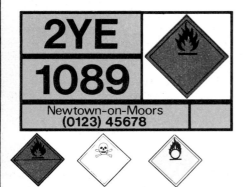

| Inflammable substances | Poisonous substances | Substances liable to ignite spontaneously |
| Radioactive substances | Corrosive substances | Compressed gases |

Fires

Rapid and clear thinking is vitally important when dealing with fires for your own sake and that of any casualties. Fire spreads very quickly so alert the emergency services immediately giving them as much information as possible. Then, try to get everyone out of the building and make sure that all doors of rooms where there is a fire are shut. *Remember, do not attempt to fight a fire unless you have notified the emergency services and have made sure that you will not be in any danger.*

Modern furniture often contains synthetic materials which, when burning, may give off toxic fumes. So you should never enter a burning building you suspect contains poisonous fumes unless equipped with, and practised in the use of, breathing apparatus. If for any reason you do have to enter a smoke-filled room, make sure you are not endangering yourself and follow the procedure described opposite.

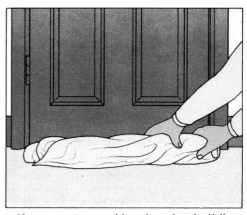

If you are trapped in a burning building, the best thing to do is to go into a room with a window and shut the door. Put a blanket or carpet against the bottom of the door to keep the smoke out and call for help from the window.

NB All the above principles apply if you are involved in a incident where there is a gas leak.

RESCUING A CASUALTY FROM A GAS OR SMOKE-FILLED ROOM

1 Check to make sure you are not in any danger.

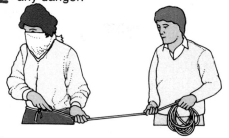

2 Rig up a life-line with a bystander and work out a system of signals so that you can be pulled to safety if necessary. The best method is to tie a rope around your waist and keep tension on the rope with a steady pull. If the tension is released, the back-up person will know you need to be pulled out.

3 Tie a wet handkerchief or scarf over your mouth and nose to keep some of the smoke out.

NB This device will *not* protect you in areas containing poisonous gas or other fumes.

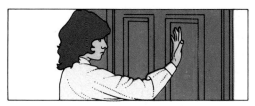

4 Feel the temperature of the door with the back of your hand and check the temperature of the air coming from under the door. If either is hot *do not* enter.

5 If it is safe to enter the room, take several deep breaths so that your blood is fully oxygenated. Then, with your shoulder at right angles to the door, open the door slightly averting your face as you do so. The room may be filled with "superheated" air under pressure which could explode.

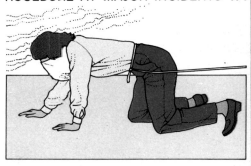

If the smoke is very dense, crawl along the floor where there should be a layer of clear air; hot air rises.

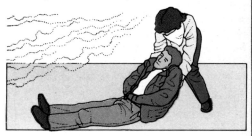

6 Locate the casualty and drag to safety as quickly as possible. Smother any smouldering clothing with a blanket, rug or coat (see p. 136).

7 If the casualty is conscious, watch very carefully. For example, where there is a smouldering fire carbon monoxide will be present in the air and this may affect the casualty's alertness.

8 If the casualty has stopped breathing, begin Artificial Ventilation immediately (see p. 18).

9 Arrange removal to hospital.

If the casualty is trapped in a garage with the car engine running, open the garage doors to ensure a good supply of fresh air. Do not attempt to enter the area until you are certain that you will not endanger yourself by doing so.

DRESSINGS AND BANDAGES

The type of dressings and/or bandages used and the techniques for applying them vary according to the type of injury sustained and the materials available. Supplies of both dressings and bandages can be bought, the former will be in sterile packs. However, substitutes can be made from household linen or any other clean non-fluffy material that is available. **NB** Fluffy material should *never* be placed directly on to a wound because the fibres will adhere.

DRESSINGS

A dressing is a protective covering which is placed on a wound to help control bleeding, prevent infection and absorb any discharge.

All dressings should be large enough to cover the area of the wound and extend about 2.5 cm (1 in) beyond it. They should, if possible, be sterile so as not to introduce germs (bacteria) which could cause infection. A dressing should also be absorbent because, if sweat cannot evaporate, the skin around the wound will become moist and the dressing sodden. This will encourage the growth of bacteria and prevent healing.

Dressings help the blood to clot thus assisting the healing process. Although a dressing may stick to a wound, making it difficult to remove later, the benefits of a dressing outweigh any damage done on removal. If a dressing becomes stained by blood immediately, do not take it off, but cover it with another dressing or dressings, as necessary.

GENERAL RULES FOR APPLYING DRESSINGS

● If possible, wash your hands thoroughly before applying dressings.

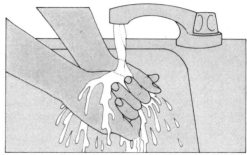

● If a wound is not too large and bleeding is under control, clean it and the surrounding skin before applying the dressing (see p. 67).
● Avoid touching the wound or any part of the dressing which will be in contact with a wound.
● Never talk or cough over a wound or the dressing.
● If necessary, cover non-adhesive dressings with pads of cotton wool to help control bleeding and absorb discharge. These pads should extend well beyond the dressing and be held in position by a bandage (see p. 177).
● If a dressing slips off a wound before you are able to secure it, renew the dressing — the first one may have picked up germs from the surrounding skin.
● Always place a dressing directly on to a wound, *never* slide it on from the side.

Adhesive Dressings

Commonly known as "plasters", these dressings consist of an absorbent gauze or cellulose pad held in place by an adhesive backing. The best have a water-repellent adhesive backing which allows moisture to evaporate from the skin. *Waterproof* plasters should *only* be used by food handlers and should not be left on for more than a few hours.

All plasters are supplied in sterile wrappings and they are available in a variety of shapes and sizes.

Always make sure the skin around a wound is clean and dry before applying an adhesive dressing otherwise it will not stick (see p. 67).

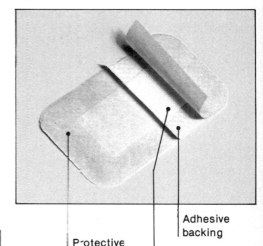

Protective layer

Gauze

Adhesive backing

Method

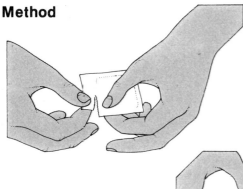

1 Remove the outer wrapping and hold the dressing, gauze-side down, by the protective strips.

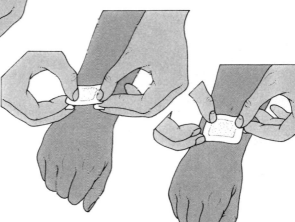

2 Peel back, but do not remove, the protective strips and, without touching the gauze, place the pad on to the wound.

3 Carefully pull off the protective strips and press the ends and the edges down.

Sterile Unmedicated Dressings

These consist of a dressing made up of layers of fine gauze and a pad of cotton wool attached to a roller bandage.

Sterile dressings are the preferred First Aid dressings for large wounds. If available, they should be used in preference to any other type of combination dressing and/or bandage on any wound. Made in a variety of shapes and sizes, sterile dressings are always enclosed and sealed in protective wrappings. *Do not use a sterile dressing if the seal is broken*.

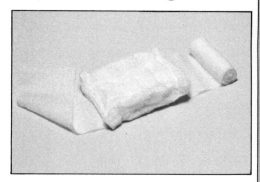

Method

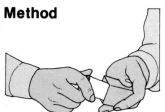

1 Remove the outer wrapping by twisting or pulling apart the outer package and remove the inner wrapping. Alternatively, pull back the tab at the end of the box and remove the inner wrapping.

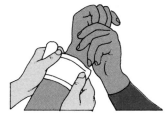

3 Hold both ends of the bandage with the folded dressing gauze-side down and over the wound; open out the dressing. If necessary, control it by placing your thumbs on the edge of the dressing, then place it on the wound.

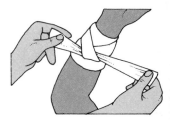

5 Secure the bandage by tying the two ends over the pad using a reef knot (see p. 180).

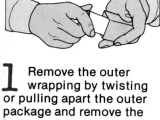

2 Holding the folded dressing and rolled bandage in one hand, unwind the short end of the bandage with the other hand.

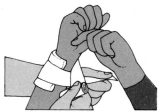

4 Wind the short end of the bandage once around the limb and dressing to secure it. Then bandage firmly until the pad is covered (see p. 186)

Gauze Dressings

These consist of layers of gauze which form a soft, pliable covering for large wounds. Gauze dressings are used if only a light covering is needed, on a burn for example, or where no sterile unmedicated dressings are available. If used instead of a sterile dressing, you should cover the gauze with a pad of cotton wool and secure it with adhesive strapping or, if pressure is required, a bandage.

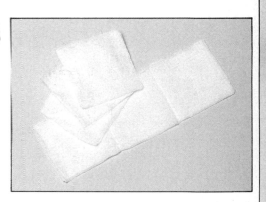

Method

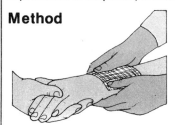 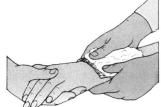 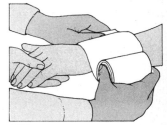

1 Remove the outer wrapping. Hold the dressing by the edges over the wound; lower it into place.

2 If necessary, cover the gauze with one or two layers of cotton wool.

3 Secure the pad with a bandage or adhesive strapping.

Adhesive Strapping

If bandages are not available or they are ineffective or difficult to apply, lengths of special adhesive strapping can be used to secure non-adhesive dressings to wounds. Adhesive strapping is available in a variety of lengths and widths.

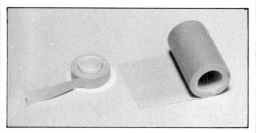

Improvised Dressings

In some emergencies prepared dressings may not be available and you will have to improvise using whatever suitable materials are to hand. Any dry, clean, absorbent material, such as the inside of a clean handkerchief, a freshly-laundered towel or piece of linen or a pad of clean paper handkerchiefs can be used. Do not place cotton wool, lint, woolly or fibrous material directly on a wound; the fibres can become embedded in it.

Improvised dressings should be covered and held in position using whatever materials are available at the time, for example, a folded scarf.

COLD COMPRESSES

Closed injuries such as bruises and sprains must be cooled to minimise swelling and relieve pain. This is best achieved by placing the injured area under cold running water. However, if the injury is on an awkward part of the body such as the head or chest or prolonged application is required, a cold compress in the form of a cold-water pack or an ice bag may have to be used instead.

APPLYING A COLD-WATER PACK

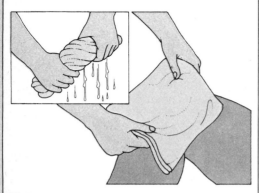

1 Soak a pad of cotton wool, towelling or similar cloth in cold or iced water. Squeeze or wring it out so that it is damp but not dripping, and place it on the injury.

2 To ensure that the cooling effect is maintained, replace pad with a fresh cold-water pack or drip more cold water on to the old one. Continue cooling the injury for 30 minutes.

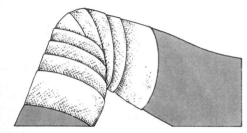

3 If necessary, cover the water pack with an open-weave bandage to hold it in position.

APPLYING AN ICE BAG

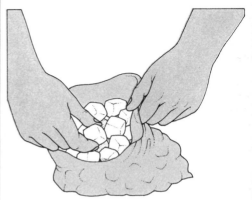

1 Fill a plastic or similar non-porous bag ½ to ⅔ full of crushed or cubed ice; add a little salt to lower the melting temperature of the ice. Exclude all air from the bag, seal it and wrap it in a cloth.

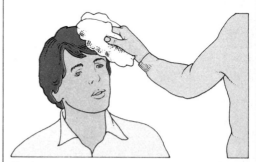

2 Place the bag over the injury; replace as necessary. Continue cooling the injury for at least 30 minutes.

3 If necessary, cover the ice bag with an open-weave bandage to hold it in position.

BANDAGES

Bandages are used to maintain direct pressure over a dressing in order to: control bleeding; hold dressings or splints in position; prevent swelling; provide support for a limb or joint; restrict movement; and, occasionally, to assist in lifting or carrying casualties. They should *not* be used for padding when other softer materials are available.

Prepared bandages are made from cotton, calico, elastic net, special paper or other materials. They are of two main types, triangular bandages and roller bandages. In an emergency, bandages can be improvised from any of the above materials or by using tights or stockings, ties, scarves or belts.

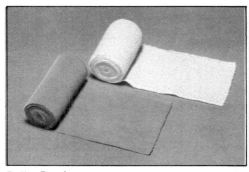

Roller Bandage

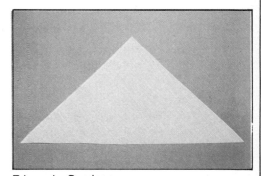

Triangular Bandage

GENERAL RULES FOR APPLYING BANDAGES

● Apply bandages when a casualty is sitting or lying down.

● Always try to sit or stand in front of the casualty and work from the casualty's injured side.

● Before you start bandaging, make sure the injured part is well-supported in the position in which it is to remain.

● If the casualty is lying down, pass all bandages under the natural hollows of the ankles, knees, back and neck. To ease them into position, gently pull them backwards and forwards and move them up or down the body.

● Bandages should be firm enough to hold the dressing in position, control bleeding or prevent movement, but not so tight that they interfere with the circulation (see *Checking Circulation* p. 178).

● Make frequent checks to ensure bandages are not becoming too tight as the tissues swell.

● Where a limb is involved ensure that the fingernails or toe-nails are exposed so that they can be checked for circulation (see overleaf).

● If a bandage is used to control bleeding and maintain direct pressure, tie the knot over the pad or dressing.

● If using bandages to immobilise a limb or part of the body, tie knots in front on the uninjured side of the body unless otherwise specified. If both sides of the body are injured, tie the knots in the centre of the body.

● When using a knot to secure a bandage *always* use a reef knot.

● Always add plenty of padding between the limbs and the body and between the limbs at the bony areas (e.g., the knees and ankles). Pay particular attention to the natural hollows (e.g., the armpits and the thighs), before applying slings and bandages.

Checking Circulation

Immediately after applying a bandage, and at 10-minute intervals thereafter, it is important to check that the circulation and/or nerves have not been interfered with by the bandage. This can be checked as indicated below and, if any of the symptoms and signs are present, adjust or remove the bandage as necessary.

Symptoms and Signs of Affected Circulation

- Casualty experiences tingling or lack of feeling in fingers or toes.
- Casualty is unable to move fingers or toes.
- Casualty's finger or toe-nail beds are unusually pale or blue.
- Pulse is absent or weak in injured limb compared to that of uninjured limb.
- Casualty's fingers/toes are very cold.

Method

Press one of the nails of the bandaged limb until it turns white. When pressure is released, the nail bed should quickly become pink again, showing that blood has returned.

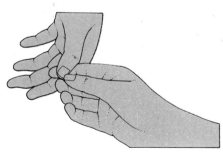

If the nail remains white or blue or the fingers are unnaturally cold, the bandage is too tight.

If no pulse can be felt in the affected limb, the bandage is too tight.

Triangular Bandages

These can be made by cutting a piece of material (linen or calico) not less than 1 m (1 yd) square in half diagonally. Alternatively, they can be bought, in which case they may be wrapped in sterile packages.

Triangular bandages can be used in a number of ways. Open or unfolded bandages can be used as a sling to provide support or protection for the arms or chest or for securing dressings over areas such as the head, hand and foot. Alternatively, they can be folded according to specific requirements (see broad and narrow bandages opposite).

STORING TRIANGULAR BANDAGES

When not in use, Triangular Bandages should be folded neatly and stored away.

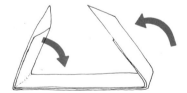

1 Make a Narrow Bandage as in steps 1 and 2 opposite.

2 Turn the ends of the bandage into the middle.

3 Continue folding the ends into the middle until a convenient size is reached.

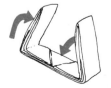

Parts of the Triangular Bandage

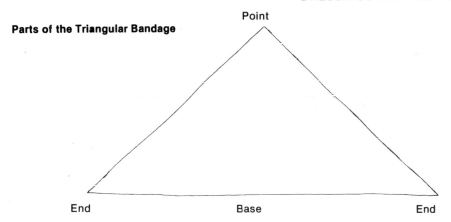

Point

End   Base   End

BROAD BANDAGES

These folded triangular bandages are used for immobilising limbs during transportation or for securing splints.

Method

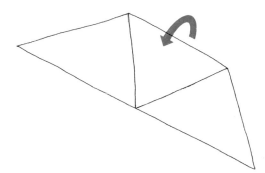

1 Turn in a narrow hem along the base of the bandage and fold the point in towards the base.

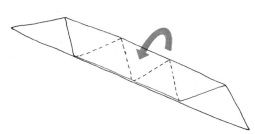

2 Fold the whole bandage in half again in the same direction.

NARROW BANDAGES

These are useful for securing a dressing at a joint if no other bandage is available (e.g., around the ankle or wrist); for applying a figure-of-eight bandage around the feet and ankles when immobilising a fractured leg (see p. 124); and for making a ring pad.

Method

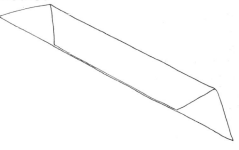

1 Make a broad bandage as in steps 1 and 2, left.

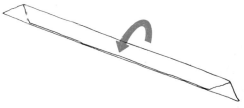

2 Fold the broad bandage in half again in the same direction.

RING PADS

Ring pads are used to build up protection around a wound in which there is a foreign body (e.g., glass) or a projecting bone (see p. 110).

Method

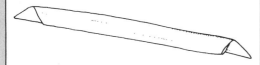

1 Make a narrow bandage, as shown on p. 179 and place it across the fingers of one hand.

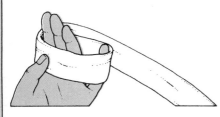

2 Wind one end once or twice around your fingers to make a loop.

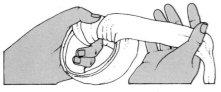

3 Bring the other end of the bandage through the loop, wind it once around the loop and pull it tight.

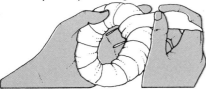

4 Working around the loop, continue passing the end through, until the whole of the bandage is used up, making a firm ring. Tuck in the end.

REEF KNOTS

Always secure the ends of a bandage with a reef knot because. it will not slip, it lies flat and is therefore more comfortable for the casualty, and is easy to untie. Once the knot is tied, the ends should be tucked out of sight or neatly fastened to the bandage. Make sure that the knot does not press on to a bone or into the skin at the back of the neck when used on a sling. If the knot is uncomfortable, place some soft material under it for padding.

Method

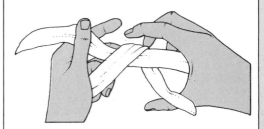

1 Take one end of the bandage in each hand. Carry the left end over the right, and under.

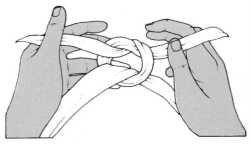

2 Bring the ends up again. Carry the right end over the left and under. Pull the knot tight and carefully tuck the ends in.

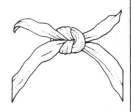

Slings

Slings are used to provide support and protection for injured arms, wrists and hands or for immobilising an upper limb when there are chest injuries. There are two types, the *Arm* sling and the *Elevation* sling. Always apply slings from the injured side so that you can provide extra support and protection.

ARM SLING

This sling is used where there are injuries to the upper limb and for some chest injuries. It holds the forearm across the chest but it is only effective if the casualty sits or stands.

When an arm sling is in the correct position the casualty's hand will be slightly higher than the elbow. The base of the bandage should lie at the root of the little finger, leaving all fingernails exposed.

Method

1 Ask the casualty to sit down and support the forearm on the injured side with the wrist and hand a little higher than the elbow — the casualty may be able to support own arm.

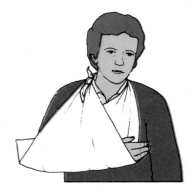

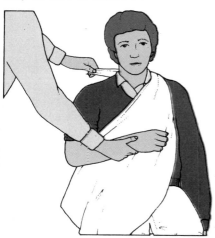

2 Using the hollow between the elbow and the chest slide one end of the triangular bandage between the chest and forearm so that its point reaches well beyond the elbow.

3 Place the upper end over the shoulder on the sound side and around the back of the neck to the front on the injured side.

4 Still supporting the forearm, carry the lower end of the bandage up over the hand and forearm and, using a reef knot, tie off on the injured side in the hollow above the collar-bone.

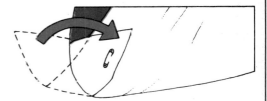

5 Finally, bring the point forward and secure it to the front of the bandage with a safety pin.

6 Check the circulation. If it is affected, adjust the bandage and/or the position of the sling.

ELEVATION SLING

This sling is used to support the hand and forearm in a well-raised position if the hand is bleeding, there are complicated chest injuries or there are shoulder injuries.

Method

1 Ask the casualty to sit down and support the injured limb. Place the forearm across the chest with the fingertips almost resting on the opposite shoulder.

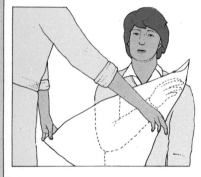

2 Place an open bandage over the forearm and hand with its point reaching well beyond the elbow and its upper end on the shoulder on the sound side.

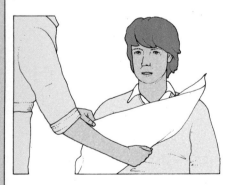

3 Still supporting the forearm, ease the base of the bandage round under the hand, forearm and elbow.

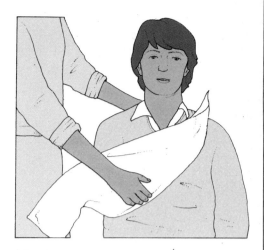

4 Carry the lower end round across the back and over to the front of the uninjured shoulder.

5 Gently adjust the height of the sling, if necessary, and, using a reef knot, tie off on the sound side in front of the hollow above the collar-bone.

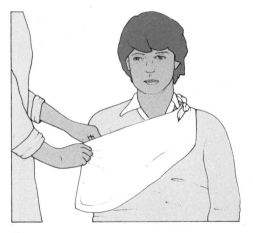

6 Tuck the point in between the forearm and the front part of the bandage. Turn the fold back against the arm and secure it with a safety pin.

7 Check the circulation. If it is affected, adjust the bandage and/or the position of the sling.

IMPROVISED SLINGS

If no triangular bandages are available, slings may be improvised in several ways to provide support.

- Support the injured limb in the fastening of a jacket or waistcoat.

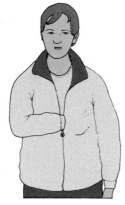

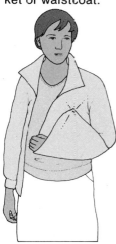

- Turn up the lower edge of the casualty's jacket and pin it to the clothing.

- Pin the sleeve of the injured limb to clothing.

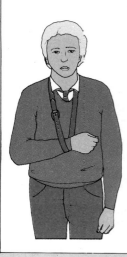

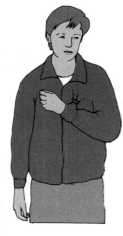

- Use a scarf, belt, tie or tights to support the limb.

Hand/Foot Bandage

This is used for holding a light dressing on to a hand or foot injury such as a graze or burn where pressure is not required. For bandaging a bleeding wound in the palm of the hand, see p. 78.

Method

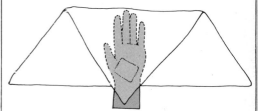

1 Keeping the injury uppermost, place a bandage under the casualty's hand with the base at the casualty's wrist and the point away from the casualty. Bring the point up over the hand to the wrist.

NB For a small hand or foot you may need to fold in a hem along the base of the bandage.

2 Carry the ends around the hand, cross them and finally, tie off below the point using a reef knot.

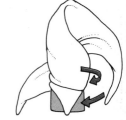

3 Bring the point down over the knot and secure.

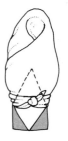

4 Check the circulation.

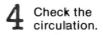

Scalp Bandage

This is used to hold dressing in place over a scalp wound but it is *not* used to control bleeding.

Method

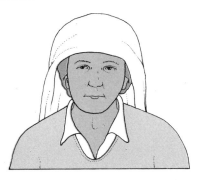

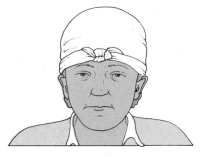

1 Fold in a hem along the base of a triangular bandage. Place the base on the forehead so that the centre of the base is above, but close to, the eyebrows and the point hangs down at the back of the head.

2 Carry the ends round to the back of the head passing just above the ears.

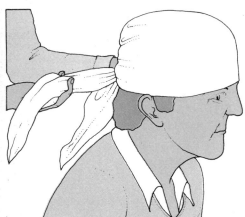

3 Cross the ends above the point of the bandage in the nape of the neck and bring them around to the front.

4 Using a reef knot tie off on the forehead close to the hem.

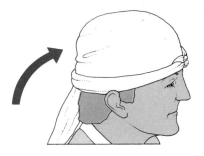

5 Steady the head with one hand and with the other, gently draw the point of the bandage down to take up the slack.

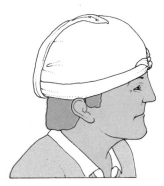

6 Turn up the point, and secure with a safety pin to the bandage on top of the head.

Roller Bandages

This type of bandage can be used to keep dressings in position, to apply pressure to control bleeding or to support a sprain or strain. Standard roller bandages are made of cotton, gauze or linen and are usually supplied in 5 m (5 yd) rolls. "Conforming" bandages hold dressings lightly but firmly in place and, because the mould to the shape of the limb, they maintain an even pressure.

Roller bandages are available in many different sizes. The size and type used will vary according to the part of the body to be bandaged and the size of the casualty (see chart below for details of sizes).

Before applying a roller bandage make sure it is tightly rolled and of a suitable width. Position yourself in front of the injury and support the injured part by hand in the position in which it is to remain. Hold the bandage with the "head" uppermost and unroll only a few inches

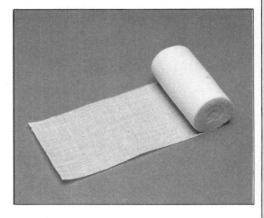

of the bandage at a time. To bandage a left limb hold the bandage in the right hand. To bandage a right limb hold it in the left hand. Always work from the inner side outwards, and from below the injury upwards.

Average Sizes of Roller Bandages for Use on Adult Casualties	
Part to be bandaged	Width
FINGER	2.5 cm (1 in)
HAND	5 cm (2 in)
ARM	5 or 6 cm (2 or 2½ in)
LEG	7.5 or 9 cm (3 or 3½ in)
TRUNK	10 or 15 cm (4 or 6 in)

Parts of a Roller Bandage

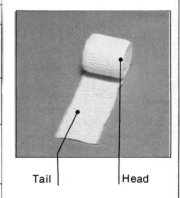

Tail | Head

When partly unrolled, the roll is called the head and the unrolled part the free end, or tail.

Applying a Roller Bandage

The most common method of applying a roller bandage is to use simple spiral turns as shown below.

Method

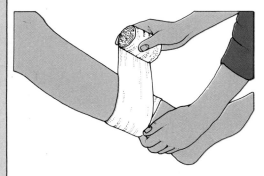

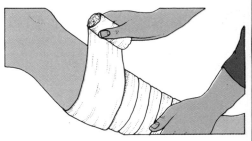

1 Begin by placing the tail of the bandage on the limb and make a firm oblique turn to hold it in position.

2 Make a series of spiral turns working up the limb. Allow each successive turn to cover two-thirds of the previous layer and leave the free edges parallel.

3 Finish off with a straight turn and secure the end.

4 Check the circulation.

Securing a Roller Bandage

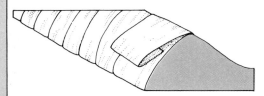

1 Finish off above the dressing. Fold in the end of the bandage.

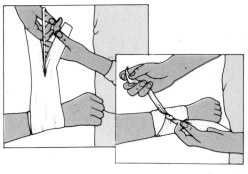

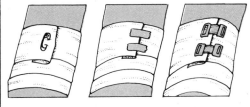

2 Secure with a safety pin, adhesive tape or a bandage clip.

If pins, tape or clips are not available, gauze bandages can be tied. Leave about 15 cm (6 in) or more of the bandage free – the amount you leave will depend on the size of the part being bandaged – and split it down the centre. Tie a knot at the bottom of the split and using a reef knot tie the ends around the limb.

Bandaging Around a Foreign Body or Open Fracture

Great care should be taken when bandaging around a foreign body or open fracture, not to apply pressure on the protrusion. Always use a roller bandage, if available. If a roller bandage is not available, a triangular bandage can be used.

Method

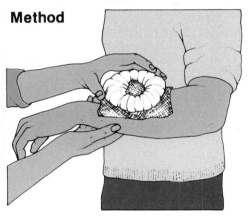

1 Drape a piece of gauze over the foreign body or fracture site and hold it in place with a ring pad or crescent-shaped pads of cotton wool (see p. 66).

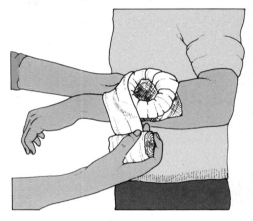

2 Place the tail of the bandage on the limb directly under the lower edge of the ring pad, make two straight turns to secure the bandage and bring the head up to the top of the pad again.

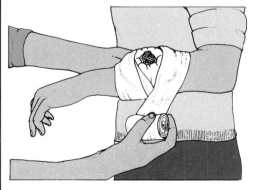

3 Pass the bandage diagonally under the limb and up over the upper half of the ring pad avoiding the protrusion. Pass the bandage back down to the start again. Continue bandaging above and below the ring pad until the pad is secure.

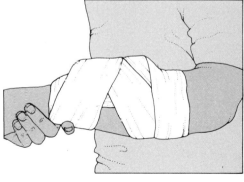

If bandaging around an open fracture wound, place the tail of the bandage on the lower part of the ring pad and make the diagonal turns *above* and *below* the ring pad to avoid pressure on the underside of the fracture.

Elbow/Knee Bandage

The method for bandaging an elbow can be adapted for bandaging a knee.

Method

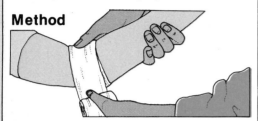

1 Ask the casualty to support the limb in the most comfortable position. Place the tail of the bandage on the inside of the elbow and make one straight turn, carrying the head over the tip of the elbow and around the limb.

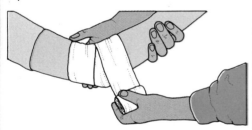

2 Take the bandage around the upper arm, covering half of the first turn, then around the forearm, covering the other edge of the first turn and touching the edge of the second turn.

3 Continue turns alternately above and below the first turn, allowing each to cover a little more than two-thirds of the previous turn.

4 Finish off with one or two spiral turns above the elbow and secure the end.

5 Check the circulation.

Hand/Foot Bandage

The method for bandaging a hand can also be used for bandaging a foot.

Method

1 Ask the casualty to support the hand with the palm held downwards. Fix the tail of the bandage at the wrist by making one straight turn.

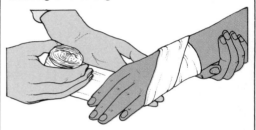

2 Carry the head of the bandage diagonally across the back of the hand towards the base of the little finger, then take it around the palm of the hand under the fingers to the base of the fingernails.

3 Carry the head of the bandage up across the top of the fingers to the root of the nail of the little finger. Then, bring it down around the palm again and diagonally across the back of the hand towards the wrist.

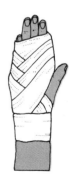

4 Continue making these figure-of-eight turns until the hand is covered. Finish off by making a spiral turn at the wrist and secure the end.

5 Check the circulation.

Tubular Gauze Bandage

Made of a roll of seamless gauze, these bandages are in many ways easier and quicker to apply than traditional bandages. They are, however, more expensive and require a special applicator.

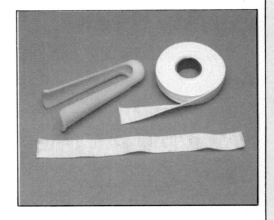

Method

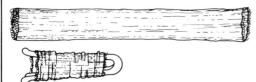

1 Cut a length of the tube gauze approximately two and a half times the length of the area to be covered. Then push the whole length of the gauze on to the applicator.

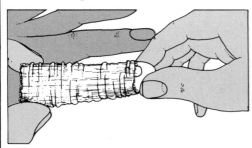

2 Gently push the applicator over the dressing on the finger. Holding the end of the gauze in position with one hand, gently pull back the applicator with the other, leaving the length of tube gauze in position on the limb.

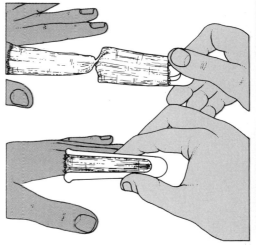

3 Holding the end of the gauze on the limb, pull the applicator back slightly, twist once or twice, and push it back on to the limb again. Withdraw the applicator leaving two layers of the gauze on the finger.

Do Not twist the gauze more than twice as you may impede the circulation.

4 Secure the end of the gauze with adhesive strapping.

SPLINTS

These are used to hold fractured or injured limbs, and sometimes the whole body, steady while a casualty is being removed to hospital. Ideally a sound leg can be used to support an injured one by tying bandages around both limbs. This is called "body-splinting". However, if this is not possible, or greater support is required for a long and/or rough journey, then a splint will be needed.

The basic requirement of any splint is that it is long enough to extend well beyond the joints above and below the injury and that it is well-padded. When placed against a limb, extra padding should be inserted where the bones touch it (e.g., at the ankles), and in the natural hollows (e.g., under the knees). For information on when and how to use splints, see *Fractures* pp. 122 – 127.

There are many different types of splints available commercially, examples are the inflatable, foam plastic, wood and wire-cage splints. Splints, however, can be improvised by using any material which is rigid, and long and broad enough to support the injured limb. Examples of this are boards, fencing pieces, sticks, brooms and rolled-up newspapers.

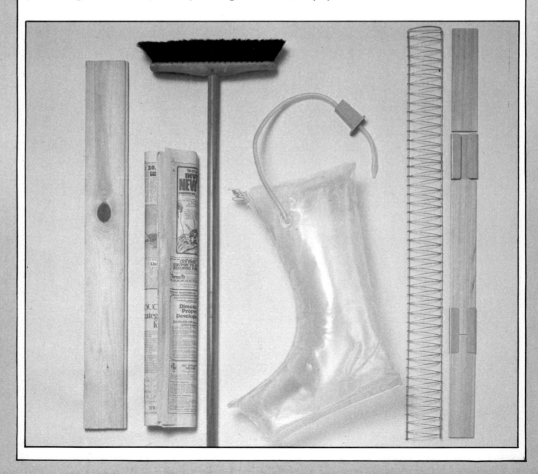

FIRST AID KITS

While bandages and dressings can be improvised it is far better to have proper equipment on hand. These materials should always be kept in a clean, dry, airtight container. Do not keep the container in a damp atmosphere such as a bathroom, and make sure that it is clearly labelled.

Below is a suggested list of contents for a first aid kit. This should be taken as a guide to the minimum you should have in a kit although you may add to the list if you wish. For example, it may be considered advisable to keep extra triangular bandages and several 25 g (1 oz) packs of cotton wool. Tweezers and scissors may also be useful.

A First Aid Kit should include:

10 Individually wrapped adhesive dressings
1   Sterile eye pad with attachment
1   Triangular bandage
1   Sterile covering for a serious wound
6   Safety pins

3   Medium sized sterile unmedicated dressings
1   Large sterile unmedicated dressing
1   Extra large sterile unmedicated dressing

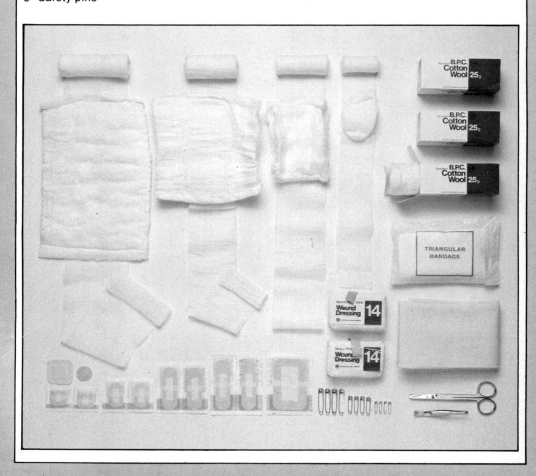

HANDLING AND TRANSPORT

The comfort, safety and well-being of the casualty are among your primary considerations and you must always make sure that the condition will not be made worse by careless handling or movement. The most important rule to remember is that you should *never move a severely injured or ill person unless there is immediate danger to life or if skilled help is not readily available*. It is better to leave the casualty undisturbed, send for help and provide First Aid treatment on the spot.

If the casualty's life is endangered by fire, falling debris or poisonous gases, move the casualty as quickly as possible without endangering yourself. Otherwise it is important, particularly if the casualty is unconscious, to carry out a quick examination before attempting to move the casualty (see pp. 36 – 40).

There are various methods of carrying casualties using support from one or more helpers, such as hand-seats and chair carries, blanket lifts and stretchers. The method used depends on: the nature and severity of the injury; the number of helpers and the facilities available; the casualty's build; the distance to shelter; and the route to be travelled.

Never attempt to move a seriously injured casualty on your own if help is available. Always make sure that everyone involved, including the casualty, if conscious, knows exactly what is going to happen and what they must do before you begin and always give a preparatory word of command before each stage.

If the casualty is to be removed to hospital you should arrange for an ambulance, although, if the injuries are minor or only involve upper limb injuries, the casualty can be taken in a car. Whichever method of transport is used, the aim is always the same — to enable the casualty to reach the destination without deterioration or discomfort. Wherever possible, the position in which the casualty is found or has been placed should not be changed and the general condition watched carefully throughout.

LIFTING CASUALTIES

This is a skill and, if it is done correctly, even a very heavy casualty can be lifted without undue strain. However, it is important that you should not attempt to lift too heavy a weight and that you always obtain assistance from any available bystanders to avoid injury to yourself.

There are two principles of lifting: first, you should always use the most powerful muscles of the body, the thigh, hip and shoulder; second, the weight should be kept as close to your body as possible.

It is very important that the correct posture for lifting is adopted. Feet should be placed comfortably apart to ensure a stable, balanced posture and a firm stance. Keep your back straight and head erect and hold the casualty close to your body using your shoulders to support the weight. Use your whole hand to strengthen the grasp. If the casualty begins to slip, do not injure your own back by trying to prevent the casualty falling. Let the casualty slide slowly and gently to the ground without causing more damage to the injured area.

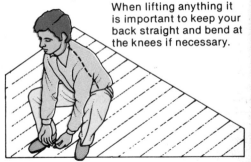

When lifting anything it is important to keep your back straight and bend at the knees if necessary.

Carries for One First Aider

If help is available, *do not* attempt to move a seriously ill or injured casualty on your own.

CRADLE METHOD
To carry lightweight casualties or children, pass one arm under the casualty's thighs and the other around the trunk above the waist and lift.

DRAG METHOD
This method involves pulling the casualty along the ground without lifting. It should *only* be used where a casualty is unable to stand and must be moved quickly from a source of danger.

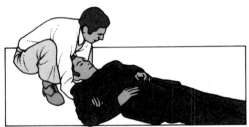

1 Fold the casualty's arms across the chest and crouch behind the casualty's head. Place your hands under the casualty's shoulders, grasp the armpits and cradle the casualty's head on your forearms.

2 Pull the casualty along the ground.

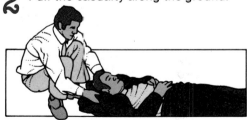

If the casualty is wearing a jacket or coat, unbutton it and pull it back up under the casualty's head. Pull the casualty along the ground in the same way with the head supported on the clothing.

HUMAN CRUTCH
This is used to support a conscious casualty who is able to walk with assistance. It should *not* be used if an upper limb is injured.

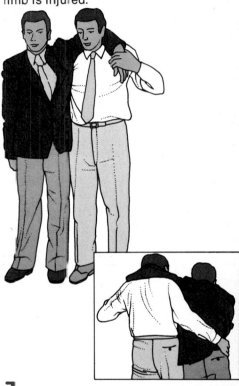

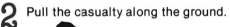

1 Stand at the casualty's injured side, if any. Place the casualty's nearest arm around your neck and hold the hand with your free hand.

2 Put your other arm around the casualty's waist and grasp the clothing at the hip. The casualty may be given additional support from a walking stick or staff.

PICK-A-BACK
If the casualty is small, light, conscious and able to hold on to you, carry in the "pick-a-back" fashion.

FIREMAN'S LIFT

This method is used to move a conscious or unconscious child or a lightweight adult when you need to keep a hand free.

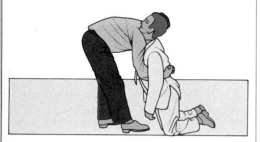

1 Help the casualty to stand up. If the casualty is unconscious or unable to stand, turn the casualty face-down and stand at the head. Place your arms under the casualty's armpits and raise the casualty on to the knees and then the feet.

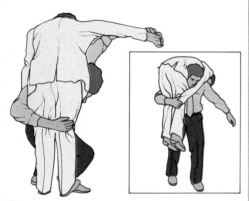

2 Grasp the casualty's right wrist with your left hand. Bend down with your head under the casualty's extended right arm so that your shoulder is level with the lower part of the abdomen; allow the casualty to fall gently across your shoulders. Place your right arm between or around the casualty's legs.

3 Taking the weight on your right shoulder stand up and gently pull the casualty across both shoulders. Transfer the casualty's right wrist to your right hand leaving your left hand free.

Carries for Two First Aiders

FOUR-HANDED SEAT

This method is used to carry a conscious casualty who can assist the bearers by using one or both arms to hold on.

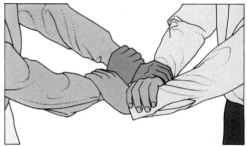

1 Stand facing each other behind the casualty. Make a seat by grasping your own left wrists with your right hands and your partner's right wrist with the free hand and stoop.

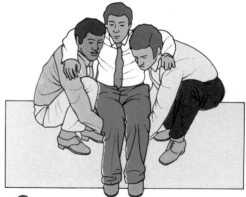

2 Instruct the casualty to place an arm around each of you at the neck, to sit back on to your hands and to steady him or herself during transport.

3 Rise together, step off with the outside feet and walk with ordinary paces.

TWO-HANDED SEAT

This method is used to carry a casualty who is unable to assist the bearers.

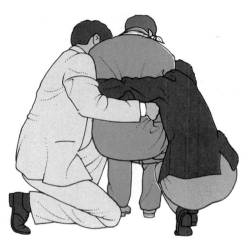

1 Squat facing each other on either side of the casualty. Each should pass the arm nearest the casualty's body under and around the back just below the shoulders and, if possible, grasp each other's wrists, otherwise, grasp the casualty's clothing.

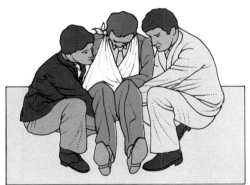

2 Raise the casualty's legs slightly, pass your other arms under the middle of the thigh and grasp each other's wrists.

3 Rise together, step off with the outside feet and walk with ordinary paces.

FORE-AND-AFT CARRY

This method can be used to place the casualty on to a chair or a carrying chair.

1 Supporting the casualty on both sides, both First Aiders should help the casualty to sit up and fold the arms across the chest.

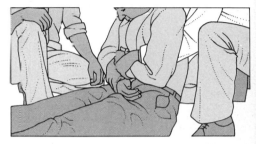

2 One person moves around behind the casualty and places the arms through and under the casualty's armpits and grasps the casualty's wrists.

Do Not use this method if you cannot grasp the casualty's wrists.

3 The other bearer remains at the casualty's side and places one arm around the casualty's back and the other under the thighs.

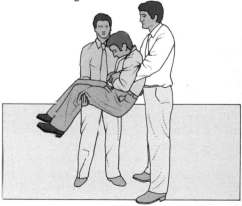

4 Working together casualty is lifted on to the chair or stretcher.

CHAIR METHOD

When a conscious casualty with no serious injuries is to be moved up or down stairs or along passageways, the casualty can be seated on an ordinary chair and carried by two people. However, the passages must be cleared of any obstructions or dangers such as loose matting before you start.

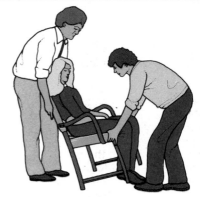

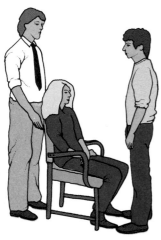

1 Test the chair to ensure that it is strong enough to support the casualty then, sit the casualty down and secure in position with broad bandages. Stand facing each other, one in front of the chair and one behind.

2 The person behind the chair should support the back of the chair and the casualty; the other should hold the chair by the front legs. Slowly tilt the chair backwards to seat the casualty securely then lift it together.

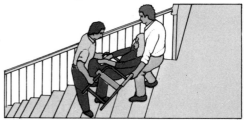

3 With the casualty facing forwards, move slowly along the passage or down the stairs.

If the stairs or passage are wide enough, you can stand facing the chair, each supporting the back and the top of a front leg of the chair.

LIFTING A CASUALTY IN A WHEELCHAIR

Wheelchair-bound casualties can be transported where they sit by adapting the chair method.

1 Locate the brakes (ask the casualty) and apply securely.

2 Sit the casualty well back in the chair.

3 Examine the wheelchair to find out which parts are fixed — arm rests and side supports are often removable and will detach if you use them to lift the chair. Supporting the chair from either side, lift by holding the fixed parts, *never* by the wheels.

4 Carry the chair as decribed above.

STRETCHERS

These are used to carry a seriously ill or injured casualty to an ambulance or similar shelter to minimise the risk of further injury. There are a variety of stretchers in general use such as: the standard stretcher; the pole-and-canvas stretcher; the Utila folding stretcher; the scoop stretcher; the carrying sheet; the carrying chair; the trolley bed; the Neil Robertson stretcher; and the paraguard stretcher.

Most stretchers can be used to transport casualties with any injury and should be rigid enough to carry casualties with suspected spine fracture without additional boards. All equipment must be tested *before* it is used.

TESTING A STRETCHER
To ensure that a stretcher is capable of taking the weight of a casualty, one person should lie on the stretcher and each end of the stretcher should be lifted in turn. Then, both ends should be lifted at the same time.

NB If possible, this should be carried out before leaving an ambulance station and not in front of a casualty.

THE STANDARD STRETCHER
The "standard" or Furley stretcher consists of poles, handles, traverses, runners and a canvas bed. The traverses are jointed so that the stretcher can be opened and closed. When closed, the poles lie close together with the canvas bed folded on top. This is then kept in position by two transverse straps. If slings are carried they are laid along the canvas held by the straps.

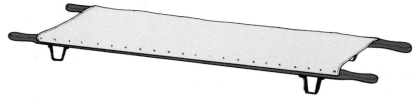

Opening the stretcher

1 Place the stretcher on its side with its runners towards you and the studs or buckles securing the straps uppermost. Unfasten any straps.

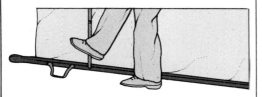

2 Push the traverses fully open with your heel and place the stretcher on its runners.

Closing the stretcher

1 Turn the stretcher on its side with its runners towards you and the studs or buckles which secure the straps uppermost. Push the joints of the traverses inwards with your heel to release them.

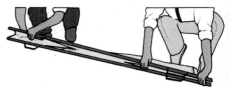

2 Push the poles together pulling the canvas out from between them. Fold the canvas neatly on to the poles and secure with the straps.

UTILA FOLDING STRETCHER

This is a lightweight version of the standard stretcher. It has light metal poles with telescopic handles and a canvas or plastic bed. The folding stretcher is available in two versions: one folds in the same way as the standard stretcher; the other folds in half in the centre and so takes up less space.

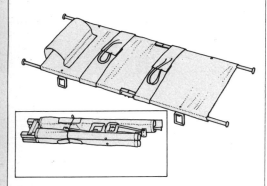

POLE-AND-CANVAS STRETCHER

This is one of the most commonly used stretchers. It consists of a canvas or plastic sheet about 200 cm (80 in) long and 50 cm (20 in) wide and two long poles. The canvas can be folded and slid under the casualty where the casualty lies (see p. 202). The poles are passed through sleeves down the side of the canvas to form the stretcher. Spacer bars may be placed over the ends of the poles to keep them apart and the stretcher firm.

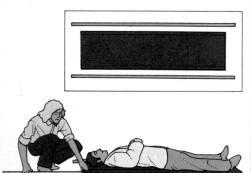

SCOOP STRETCHER

The scoop or orthopaedic stretcher is an adjustable stretcher used to lift casualties on to an ambulance trolley bed without altering the position in which they were found. It is not used to carry a casualty any distance. The length can be adjusted to suit any size of casualty and because the casualty does not have to be moved, it is particularly useful for picking up a casualty with a suspected spine fracture or internal injuries.

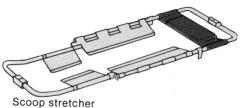

Scoop stretcher

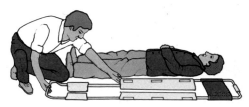

1 Bring the stretcher to the casualty's side and adjust the length.

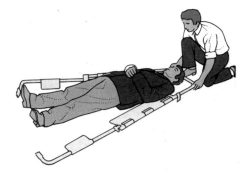

2 Uncouple both ends of the stretcher and gently slip each half of the stretcher under the casualty; rejoin the head sections.

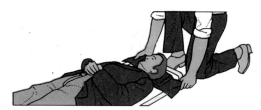

3 Place the head pad in position.

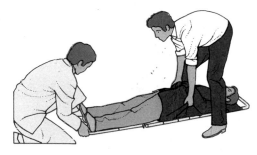

4 While one First Aider stays at the casualty's head, the other should rejoin the foot section. Secure the head pad to the stretcher.

5 Working from either side of the stretcher, lift the stretcher and casualty and place on the trolley bed. Leave the stretcher in position or uncouple and remove it if other casualties are to be moved.

TROLLEY BED

This is a fully-adjustable stretcher bed on wheels made of light metal which is carried in many ambulances.

Trolley beds should always be kept prepared for immediate use. A canvas sheet from a pole and canvas stretcher is laid on the stretcher bed and two blankets are placed on top (see p. 201).

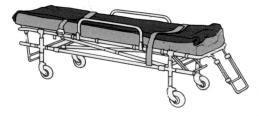

NEIL ROBERTSON STRETCHER

Made of stout canvas and bamboo this stretcher is designed for lifting casualties in the *upright* position through small hatches, such as manholes or pothole entrances, or for lowering casualties from heights as in mountain rescue.

The casualty is placed on the stretcher. Rope at the base acts as "stirrups" to hold the casualty's feet. The strap at the top is passed around the casualty's forehead to hold the head in position. The upper flaps are wrapped around the casualty's chest and secured with the two short straps, leaving the arms outside. The casualty's arms are then secured with the long strap. The lower flaps are strapped round the lower limbs.

The ring at the head of the stretcher is used for hoisting. Another length of rope is attached to the ring at the foot of the stretcher to guide the stretcher.

The stretcher should be stored in a place where it is most likely to be needed together with a suitable length of rope, preferably made of a rot-proof fibre.

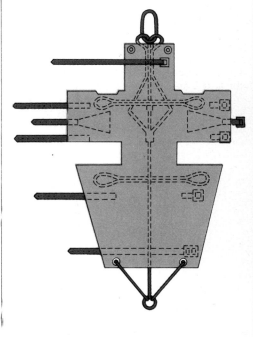

PARAGUARD STRETCHER

This stretcher is similar to the Neil Robertson stretcher and is used for the same purposes. However, it is lighter, less cumbersome and more durable than the Neil Robertson and can be folded up and carried on the back. The main advantage of the paraguard stretcher is that it will bend in the middle so you can negotiate obstacles.

IMPROVISED STRETCHERS

Stretchers may be improvised as follows:
● Turn the sleeves of two or three coats inside out. Pass two strong poles through the sleeves and button up the coats. The poles may be kept apart by

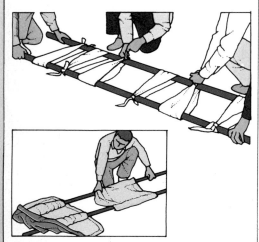

strips of wood tied to the poles at each end of the stretcher.
● Tie broad bandages at intervals around two strong poles.
● Make holes in the bottom corners of one or more sacks and pass strong poles through them; keep them apart as above.
● Spread out a rug, piece of sacking, tarpaulin or a strong blanket and roll up two strong poles in the sides
● Use a hurdle, broad piece of wood, door or shutter and add a rug, clothing, or hay or straw covered with a piece of stout cloth or sacking.
NB Always test an improvised stretcher (see Testing a stretcher p. 197).

Preparing a Stretcher or Trolley Bed

To protect and keep the casualty warm, blanket the stretcher according to the number of blankets available.

WITH ONE BLANKET

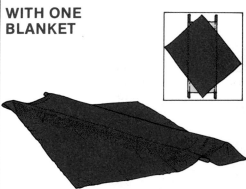

1 Place the blanket diagonally over the stretcher so that there are two opposing corners at the ends of the stretcher.

2 After placing the casualty on the stretcher, bring the point of the blanket at the foot of the stretcher up over the casualty's feet and tuck a small fold between the ankles.

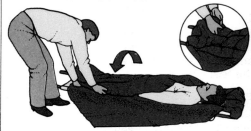

3 Fold the point of the blanket at the head around the head and neck. Bring the right side of the blanket over the casualty and tuck it in. Then bring the left side of the blanket over and tuck it in.

WITH TWO BLANKETS

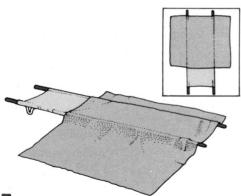

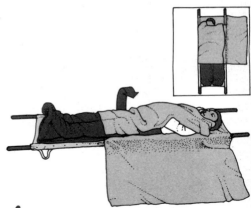

1 Place the first blanket lengthwise across the stretcher with one edge covering half the handles at the head and leaving slightly more to one side of the stretcher than the other.

4 Bring the folds of the blanket over the legs and feet and tuck them in.

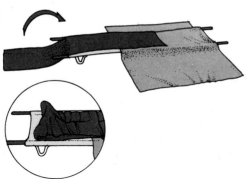

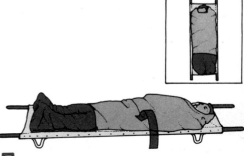

2 Fold the second blanket lengthwise into three and place on the stretcher with the upper edge about one third of the way down the stretcher leaving enough at the bottom end to fold in over the feet.

3 After placing the casualty on the stretcher bring the foot of the top blanket up over the casualty's feet and tuck a small fold between the ankles to prevent rubbing.

5 Turn in the upper corners of the first blanket and bring the shorter side over the casualty and tuck it in. Finally, bring the long side of the blanket over the casualty and tuck it in.

Loading a Stretcher

Ideally five people will be required to load a casualty on to a stretcher — four to lift the casualty and one to move the stretcher. However, there are methods of moving a casualty using two or three bearers if there are not enough people available or space is limited. The First Aider in charge of the casualty should assemble a squad of four bearers, decide which method of lifting is to be used, make it clear to each person what is to be done and give *all* the directions.

If you are unloading a stretcher in order to place a casualty on to a bed or examination couch reverse the loading procedure.

LOADING A CASUALTY ON TO A POLE-AND-CANVAS STRETCHER

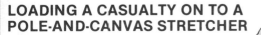

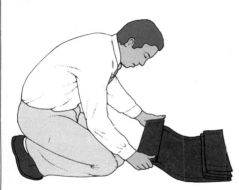

1 Working from top and bottom fold the canvas sheet into a concertina-shape; make three complete folds from the top and four from the bottom. Slide the folded canvas under the casualty through the hollow of the back.

2 Each person should place one foot on the top pile of folds, pull the casualty's clothing taut from the waist down and gently work the canvas down under the buttocks and legs. Repeat for the top part of the body until the canvas is extended.

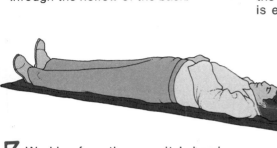

3 Working from the casualty's head, slide the poles into the sleeves and place spacer bars over the ends if they are to be used. Lift the stretcher as described on pp. 206 – 9.

PLACING A BLANKET UNDER THE CASUALTY

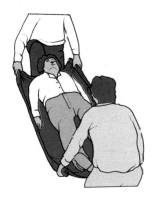

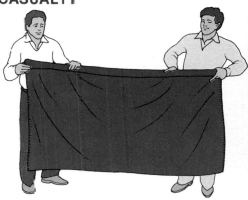

1 Test the blanket. Lay the blanket on the ground. One person should lie down on the blanket while two others attempt to lift it.

2 Roll a blanket or rug lengthwise for half its width; place the roll in line with and against the injured side of the casualty (or most severely injured side if both are injured).

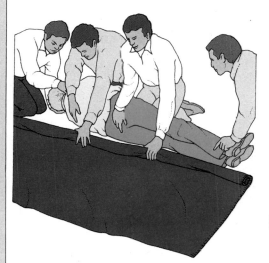

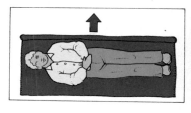

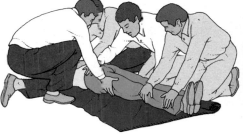

3 All four bearers should work together and turn the casualty slowly and gently on to the side away from the blanket. Move the rolled portion of the blanket or rug up against the casualty's back.

4 Gently turn the casualty on to the back over the roll of the blanket and far enough on to the opposite side to allow the blanket to be unrolled. Turn the casualty on to the back again.

NB This method can also be used to load a casualty on to a pole-and-canvas stretcher.

BLANKET LIFT

1 Stand so that two bearers face each other on either side of the trunk, and two face each other at the lower limbs. Tightly roll the two edges of the blanket up against the casualty's sides.

If poles of sufficient length and rigidity are available, the edges of the blanket can be rolled around them. It will make the casualty easier to lift and prevent the blanket sagging.

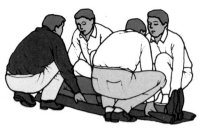

2 With backs straight, squat and grasp the blanket with palms downwards and fingers at the inner side of the rolled blanket edge. The two bearers nearest the casualty's head should each place one hand level with the head and the other at the waist. The bearers at the lower limbs should place one hand level with the hips and the other at the ankles.

3 Working together, carefully and evenly lift the casualty high enough to enable a fifth person to push the stretcher underneath.

4 Working together again, carefully and evenly lower the casualty on to the stretcher.

If a fifth person is not available or if it is not possible to push the stretcher under the casualty, place the stretcher in line with the casualty as close to the head as possible. Carefully lift the casualty and move with short even side paces until the casualty is directly over the stretcher then lower the casualty on to it.

MANUAL LIFTS

If a blanket is not available you will have to lift the casualty using one of the following methods.

For Four Bearers

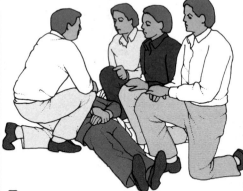

1 Three bearers should place themselves on the left of the casualty: one facing the knees, one facing the hips and the third facing the shoulders. The bearer in charge of the casualty should be on the casualty's right facing the middle bearer.

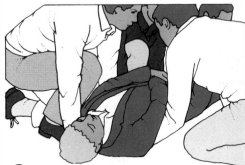

2 All bearers should go down on their left knees and place their forearms beneath the casualty paying particular attention to the site of the injury. The person in charge should grasp the left wrist of the bearer at the shoulders with the left hand and the right wrist of the bearer opposite with the right hand. The person at the shoulders should support the head and shoulders and ensure an open airway and the fourth bearer should support the lower limbs.

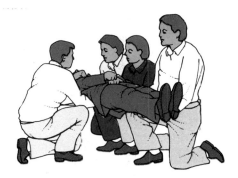

3 When the order "lift" is given by the person in charge raise the casualty gently, slowly and evenly and place on the knees of the other three bearers.

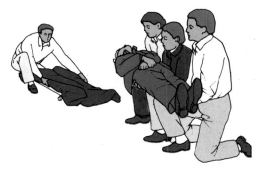

4 If a fifth person is not available to move the stretcher, the person in charge should disengage, get the prepared stretcher and place it under the casualty. It should be positioned so that the casualty's head will be just clear of the top traverse when lowered on to it. The bearer should then resume the original position and rejoin hands.

5 When the order "lower" is given, work together and gently raise the casualty slightly from the bearers' knees. Then slowly and evenly lower the casualty on to the stretcher bed.

For three bearers

1 Place the stretcher in line with the casualty as near the head as possible. One bearer should kneel on one knee on the injured side of the casualty level with the knees and place the hands under the casualty's legs. The other two should kneel on opposite sides of the casualty's chest and grasp each others' wrists under the shoulders and hips.

2 On the order "lift", gently and evenly raise the casualty and stand up. Then, moving with side paces, carry the casualty head first over the stretcher.

3 When the order "lower" is given, gently, slowly and evenly lower the casualty on to the stretcher.

If the casualty is seriously injured and must be kept rigid all three bearers should work from the same side. They should raise the casualty and tilt the body towards them as they lift.

LOADING A CASUALTY IN THE RECOVERY POSITION

1 Prepare the stretcher as on p. 200 but place one extra rolled blanket down one side of the stretcher to support the casualty in the Recovery Position.

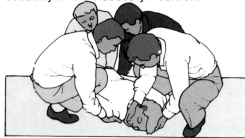

2 Bring the casualty's arms down by the side; three bearers should stand on the casualty's left at the head to ensure an open airway, at the hips and the knees while a fourth person supports the casualty's trunk from the other side.

3 Follow the procedure described left and opposite.

Carrying a Stretcher

When the casualty has been placed on the stretcher the bearers should take up their positions at each end of the stretcher. At least two trained bearers will be required to carry a stretcher and the person in charge of the casualty should always remain at the casualty's head. If bystanders are available they should be used to help carry the stretcher to spread the load. However, there should be at least one trained bearer at each end of the stretcher.

Unless a casualty is suffering from shock, the head should be kept higher than the feet. So as a general rule the casualty should always be carried feet first. However, there are a few exceptions:
- When going up stairs or hills when the lower limbs are *not* injured.

- When going down stairs or hills when the casualty's lower limbs *are* injured or the casualty is suffering from hypothermia.
- When carrying a casualty to the side or foot of a bed.
- When loading a casualty into an ambulance.

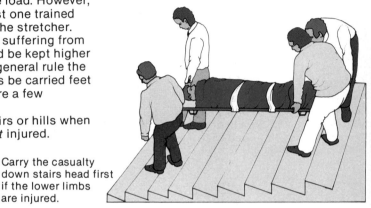

Carry the casualty down stairs head first if the lower limbs are injured.

FOR FOUR BEARERS

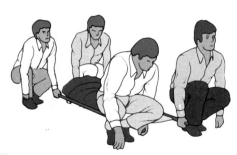

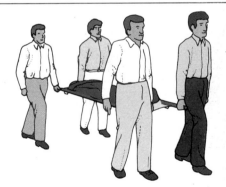

1 Keeping their backs straight, all the bearers should squat and grasp the handles with their inner hands, palms inwards. On the order "lift", all rise together, holding the stretcher with arms fully extended and keeping it level.

2 At the order "Advance", move off together but walk out of step to avoid bouncing the stretcher.

3 When you reach the ambulance, working together, gently and evenly lower the stretcher to the ground with the casualty's head nearest the ambulance.

CROSSING UNEVEN GROUND

A stretcher should, if possible, be carried by four bearers when crossing uneven ground. Secure the casualty to the stretcher with a harness or broad bandages before you start. Keep the stretcher as nearly level as possible; this can be done by each bearer adjusting the height of the stretcher individually.

If crossing very uneven ground for a short distance, the four bearers should stand at the side of the stretcher facing inwards. Grasp the poles with one hand and place the other about 75 cm (30 in) in from the end of the stretcher; then, move with side paces and *not* cross-over steps.

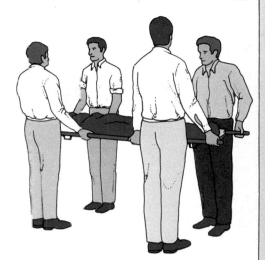

CROSSING A WALL

Always avoid crossing a wall, if possible, even if it means carrying a stretcher further. However, if there is no gap, follow the procedure described below.

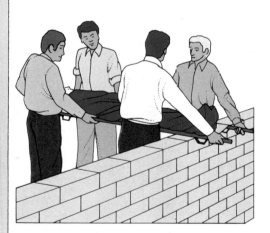

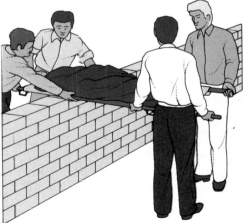

1 Lower the stretcher in front of the wall and turn inwards. Lift the stretcher and rest it on the wall, with the front runners beyond the wall.

2 The front bearers should cross the wall one at a time while the others steady the stretcher.

3 All the bearers should lift the stretcher again and move the stretcher forward until the rear runners are close to the approach side of the wall. The remaining bearers then cross the wall one at a time while the others steady the stretcher.

4 Finally, lower the stretcher to the ground then carry it in the usual way.

MOVING A STRETCHER FROM ONE LEVEL TO ANOTHER

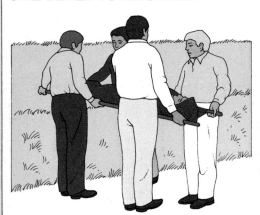

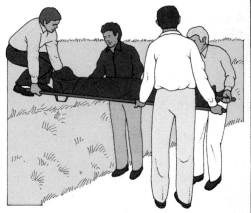

1 All the bearers should stand at the side of the stretcher as shown for crossing uneven ground (see p. 207). Lift the stretcher so that it is level with the top of the bank and place the foot of the stretcher on the bank.

2 One bearer should then get up on to the bank ready to receive the stretcher while the others move it forward.

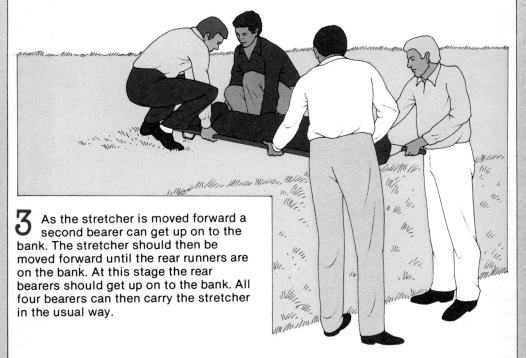

3 As the stretcher is moved forward a second bearer can get up on to the bank. The stretcher should then be moved forward until the rear runners are on the bank. At this stage the rear bearers should get up on to the bank. All four bearers can then carry the stretcher in the usual way.

Loading an Ambulance

A few ambulances have flat built-in beds with grooves to take the runners of a standard stretcher. Four people will be required to load this ambulance: one to stand inside the ambulance ready to guide the stretcher, while the other three stand one or either side of the stretcher and one at the end ready to lift. If there are two berths, always load the left one first.

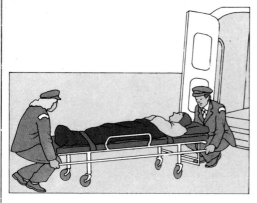

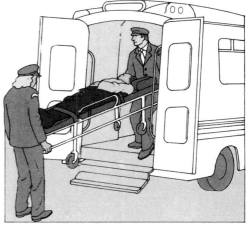

1 If loading a trolley bed into an ambulance, two bearers should take up their positions one at each end of the trolley bed.

2 Working together, raise the trolley bed to the required height and carry it head first into the ambulance.

Unloading an Ambulance

Two bearers take hold of the handles at the rear and gently withdraw the stretcher. As it is withdrawn, two more bearers may take hold of the handles at the head and, taking the weight, lower it so that their arms are fully extended. Then, moving with side-paces, carry the stretcher clear of the ambulance and lower it to the ground.

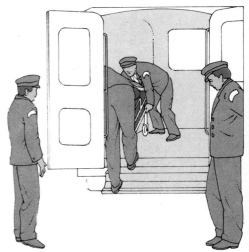

Miscarriage

A miscarriage or "spontaneous abortion" is the loss of the embryo or foetus at any time before the 28th week of pregnancy. It is usually due to abnormality or death of the foetus and is therefore a protective mechanism that avoids the full development and birth of an abnormal baby.

About 20 per cent of all pregnancies end in miscarriage. Although some women may experience a "threatened" miscarriage involving little or no pelvic pain and only slight "spotting" of blood from the vagina, complete miscarriages always include the very real danger of severe vaginal bleeding. Incomplete miscarriage is serious because products of the conception are retained in the womb and it can result in severe bleeding.

Symptoms and Signs

● Vaginal bleeding and, if severe, symptoms and signs of shock (see p. 90).

● Cramp-like pains in the lower abdomen or pelvic area; these may be severe.

● Passage of the foetus and other products of conception.

Aim

Reassure and comfort casualty and arrange removal to hospital.

Treatment

1 Reassure the casualty and keep her warm. Lay her down with head and shoulders raised and knees slightly bent.

2 Check pulse (see p. 89) and breathing rate (see p. 12).

3 Place a sanitary towel or clean towel over the vagina.

4 Remove to hospital immediately.

EMERGENCY CHILDBIRTH

A woman may go into labour unexpectedly at a time and place where she is unable to put her arrangements for confinement into practice. Also, a few women make no preparation at all.

It is important to remember that childbirth is a natural process and that the majority of births do not threaten the life of either mother or baby. In most cases, there is adequate time to arrange transport to hospital, or for the assistance of a doctor or midwife, but it is nonetheless essential that you clearly understand what you can do and what you should not do, before expert help arrives.

In a normal birth, the baby's head will emerge first. Rarely, however, the baby's position in the womb is reversed. This is known as a *Breech Birth* (see p. 216) and it requires urgent medical attention.

Never try to delay a birth in any way. Allow the delivery to proceed without interfering until the baby's head is emerging.

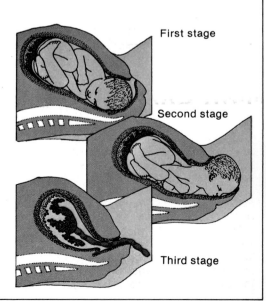

First stage

Second stage

Third stage

The First Stage

The first indication that labour has started is when the mother notices a low backache. A "show" of blood-stained mucus is a sign that the neck of the womb (cervix) has softened and dilated and the mucus plug has come away. At this stage the womb (uterus) contracts every 10 to 20 minutes, dilating the neck of the womb and the birth canal.

This stage may take 15 to 16 hours for a first child and about 10 hours for the second or any subsequent pregnancies. You should have ample time to call an ambulance and have the mother safely transported to hospital.

Towards the end of the first stage, the cramp-like contractions become more painful and more frequent. The "waters" will break indicating that the bag containing the amniotic fluid in which the baby lies has ruptured. Half a litre (1 pint) or more of liquid may escape in a sudden rush, although sometimes a constant trickle is all that is evident. When this occurs, it means that the baby is on its way, the second stage of labour has begun and the mother needs help.

The Knee-Elbow Position
Very rarely the cord protrudes into the birth canal after the waters have broken. If this occurs, place the mother in the Knee-Elbow position, to reduce pressure on the cord, and remove to hospital immediately.

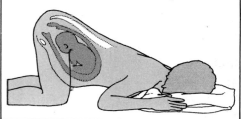

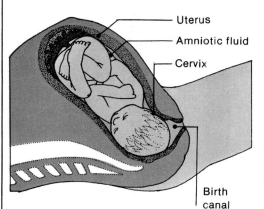

Uterus

Amniotic fluid

Cervix

Birth canal

The Second Stage

It is during this stage that the baby will be born. It generally lasts about one hour for a first baby and thirty to forty-five minutes for any subsequent births. Always remember that from the first sign of labour there is plenty of time to get ready so do not fuss.

Do not move the mother. Remain calm and if this is not already being done, immediately despatch someone to call for an ambulance. Instruct them to give the ambulance control details of the

stage of labour that has been reached, together with the name, if any, of the hospital into which the mother is booked and the address where she can be found (see *Calling for Assistance*, p. 35).

Once the contractions are approximately two minutes apart and the mother is pushing down and straining hard with contractions, she needs help immediately. It is now essential that a warm, quiet environment be arranged for the delivery of the baby.

Preparing for the Birth

The prospective mother is likely to be very nervous and excited. It is most important that she should be reassured of your ability to deal with the situation. This is best done by talking calmly to her and making the whole thing appear as an everyday occurrence.

All unnecessary people should be asked to leave the room, but make sure you are not left alone with the mother.

Usually there will be a female relative or a neighbour you can ask to help, and the father, if available, may want to stay.

Protect the bed, sofa or floor with any plastic sheeting that may be available, but remember that towels or newspaper can be used as a substitute. If the mother is not at home or near a bed, she can lie down on the floor, the seat of a car, or any flat surface. In a public place, if there

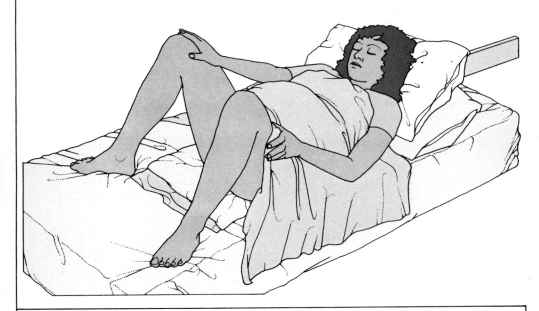

PREVENTING INFECTION

Lack of scrupulous cleanliness and infection can jeopardise the lives of both the mother and the baby. No person who has a cold, sore throat or septic hands should help with the delivery. You and your assistant should both wear masks. If none are available, you can improvise by tying clean handkerchiefs around your faces. If possible, scrub your hands, nails and forearms thoroughly under running water for four minutes. Do not dry them and if they become soiled, wash them again in the same way.

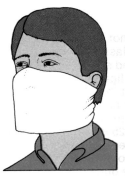

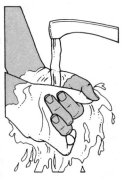

Delivery

are people around, ask them to stand with their backs to her to afford some privacy.

Lay the mother on her back with her knees drawn up and her head and shoulders comfortably supported. Ask her to remove any clothing that will interfere with the delivery. Cover her with blankets for as long as is possible and put cotton, lint or any suitable sheeting under her buttocks for warmth, and to absorb any subsequent mess. Fold a blanket in three and wrap it in a sheet to make a pack to cover the top half of her body during the delivery.

For the baby
Make sure there is some form of heating available. Prepare a cot and have a blanket, shawl or towel ready to wrap up the baby. A cot can be improvised from linen baskets, drawers or boxes. Place it in a corner away from any draughts.

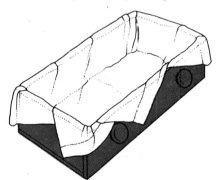

For the delivery
Fill some jugs with hot water and find a clean basin, and a plastic or stout paper bag to hold the soiled swabs, etc. Have scissors and sterile ligatures ready in case you need to cut the umbilical cord. Boil the scissors for ten minutes to sterilise them. If there are no ligatures available, boil three 25 cm (9 in) pieces of string (for ten minutes) or soak in methylated spirits (for ten minutes). You will also need sterile dressings (see p. 174) to dress the cord after cutting.

During contractions, the labouring mother, should be encouraged to grasp her knees, bend her head forward, hold her breath and push, and then to relax between contractions.

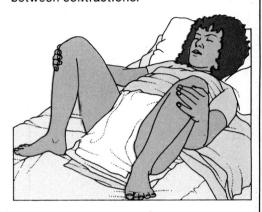

Eventually the perineum will become distended, a bulge will appear and, during the contractions, you will see the baby's head at the entrance to the birth canal — it will recede between contractions. This indicates that the birth is imminent.

More of the baby's head will appear with each contraction. You must steady the baby's head as it emerges because while in the birth canal it is subjected to great pressure during contractions. If it is allowed to "shoot out" the sudden change of pressure could rupture a blood vessel in the baby's brain. This may result in brain damage. *Do not* pull on or twist the baby's head.

Check as soon as possible whether or not the umbilical cord (a soft thick, gelatinous-looking rope) is around the baby's neck. If it is, it can usually be gently eased over the head. *Do not* pull it.

If the bag of fluid in which the baby is lying inside the mother has not broken before the birth, there may be a covering (membrane) over the baby's face as it emerges. This must be torn as soon as possible to prevent asphyxia and to allow the fluid to escape.

Procedure for delivery

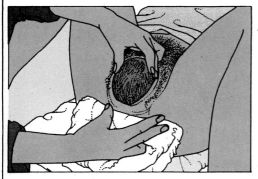

1 Place a clean pad over the back passage (anus). If a bowel movement occurs wipe it from front to back to avoid soiling the birth canal.

Do Not put your fingers into the birth canal.

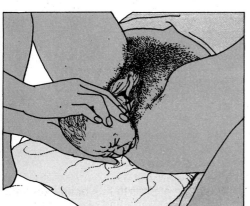

2 Gently support the baby's head as it emerges and steady it to prevent it "shooting" out.

If there is a covering over the baby's face, tear it with your fingers to prevent asphyxia.

Check the position of the umbilical cord. If it is around the baby's neck, gently ease it over the head.

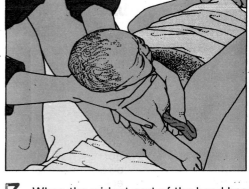

3 When the widest part of the head has passed through the birth canal, tell the mother to open her mouth and pant. Support the baby's body as it is born.

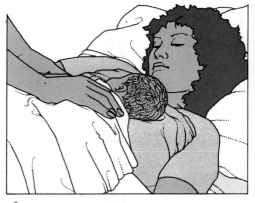

4 Once the baby is born, lift it on to the mother's abdomen and clear out its mouth (See *Care of the Newborn Baby*, opposite).

Do Not pull the cord in any way; remember that it is still attached to the mother. (There is no need to cut the cord at this stage.)

Hold the baby very carefully because it will be very slippery. Lay it down so that the head is lower than the body. Make sure the mother and baby are covered and warm.

Care of the Newborn Baby

As soon as the baby has emerged, open its mouth and wipe away any blood or fluid with a swab. By this time it will probably be crying and it is quite possible for you to clean it up a little more. Wrap up the baby in something soft and warm. Make sure that its head is pointing down, so that any fluid or mucus can drain from the mouth and nose, and ensure the airway is kept clear.

The baby can be allowed to suck at the breast if the mother desires.

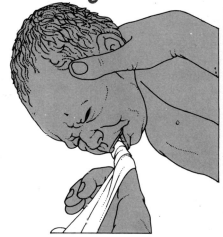

THE NON-BREATHING BABY

Occasionally, the baby does not cry and if it is not breathing, there may be an obstruction in the airway. This is usually mucus and must be cleared immediately.

1 Carefully clear the baby's airway wiping the mouth and nose.

Do Not smack the baby.

2 If the baby fails to respond and is either blue or white and completely limp then begin resuscitation immediately (see pp. 18 – 23).

The Third Stage

At any time between 10 and 30 minutes after the birth of the baby, the *afterbirth* should separate from the mother's womb. When it is about to be expelled, the mother will experience mild contractions. Encourage her to hold her breath and push the afterbirth out. She will find this easiest if she is lying down with her knees up and apart. *Do not* pull the afterbirth or cord while it is being expelled. There is no need to separate the birth from the cord, this can safely until medical aid is available. Keep preferably in a polythene bag, as be checked for complete-mother reaches hospital.

Even a small piece left inside the mother can cause complications later.

When the afterbirth has been expelled, clean up the mother and lay a sanitary towel or clean cloth over the vagina. Make her as comfortable as possible and encourage her to rest. A small amount of bleeding is normal. Severe bleeding rarely occurs, but, if this does happen, remember skilled help is on the way, so keep calm. Gently massage the mother's abdomen just below the navel to stimulate the uterus to contract. The uterus will harden as it contracts but continue massage until skilled help arrives.

Breech Delivery

This is where the baby's position in the womb is reversed. It is not a common condition but it is one which requires urgent medical attention.

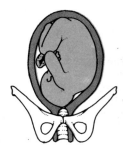
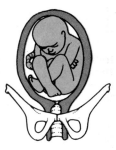

Normal (Head down)   Breech (Head up)

Treatment

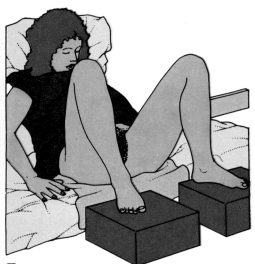

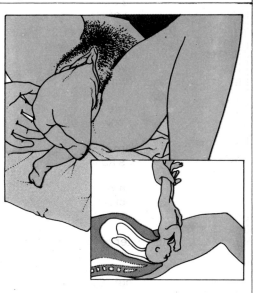

1 If the mother is on a bed, lay her across the bed with her buttocks at the edge and her legs and feet over the side. Place two boxes or stools under her feet to support the legs.

2 Gently support the baby as it appears. Keep its body warm so as not to stimulate breathing by excessive cooling before the head emerges.

3 Allow the baby to hang from the birth canal during delivery. If the head is retained for more than three minutes after the shoulders have appeared, grasp the feet and lift baby over the mother's abdomen to free mouth and nose.

4 Clean any mucus from the baby's mouth and nose to open the airway.

5 Wait for the rest of the head to emerge. Too rapid a delivery m cause brain damage, and once th and nose are free, there is no n hasten the rest of the delive

Dealing with the Cord

In most instances no harm will result if the umbilical cord is left attached to the baby until mother and baby reach hospital. If the cord is very short or removal to hospital will be delayed, it may be necessary to cut the cord. Wait until: after the afterbirth has been delivered; the cord has stopped pulsating; or until at least ten minutes after the birth.

1 Using two of the sterile ligatures, or prepared pieces of string (see p. 213), tie the cord very firmly in two places: 15 cm (6 in) and 20 cm (8 in) from the baby's abdomen. If the ligature nearest the baby is not tied very firmly the baby may bleed to death when the cord is cut.

2 Cut the cord between the two ties using sterilised scissors.

3 Place a sterile dressing over the cut end at the baby's abdomen.

Do Not put powder or disinfectant of any kind on the cut end of the cord.

4 Ten minutes after cutting, inspect the cord to make sure there is no bleeding. Tie the remaining ligature around the cord about 10cm (4 in) from the baby's abdomen.

5 Dress the cord again with another sterile dressing and secure it by tying a folded napkin around the baby.

If there is no sterile dressing available, do not tie anything around the baby.

If the cord has to be cut before the afterbirth has been expelled, cover the end of the umbilical cord attached to the afterbirth with a sterile dressing. **Always keep the afterbirth so that it can be inspected later.**

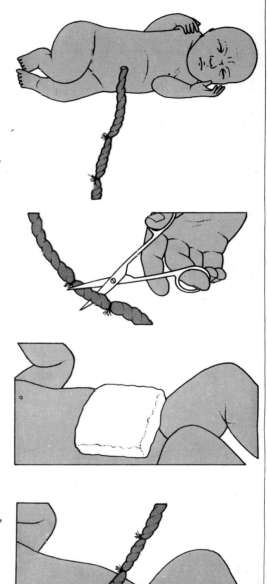

INDEX

ACKNOWLEDGMENTS

Editor Jemima Dunne

Art Director Patrick Nugent
Designers Derek Coombes, Nick Maddren

Managing Editor Amy Carroll
Managing Art Director Debbie MacKinnon

Illustrators
Russell Barnett
Will Giles
Hayward and Martin
Edwina Keene
Gary Marsh
Andrew Popkiewicz
Jim Robins
Venner Artists

Photography
All special photographs by Roger Banning; p. 167 Ian Christy/Daily Telegraph

Photographic Services
Negs Photographic Services Ltd.

Typesetting
Colset Private Ltd, Singapore
Rowland Phototypesetting, London

Reproduction
Hong Kong Graphic Arts

Dorling Kindersley would like to thank:
Dr. A. Armstrong; Dr. J.N. Blau, City of London Migraine Clinic; Daphne Crabtree; Lesley Gilbert; Andrew Gordon Craig Ph.D, British Epilepsy Association; J. Hornby; Dr. R. Langford; Chief Officer and Training School, London Ambulance Service; E.A. Malkin FRCS; Yvonne McFarlane; Dr J. Mowat; Ron Pickless; Robert Sandham, Smith and Nephew Ltd.

The Joint Revision Committee consisted of: Captain F.A. Bland, Dr. P.A.B. Raffle from St. John Ambulance; Dr. J. Junor, Dr. H. Macdonald, D. Strachan, Dr. J. Wilson from St. Andrew's Ambulance Association; Miss M. Baker, Major-General R.J. Gray from The British Red Cross Society. The committee is grateful for the assistance of Miss. J. Eaves and J. McKenzie